A Doctor's Guide to Home Medical Care

The A to Z Handbook of Common
Symptoms, Illnesses, and Emergencies

Trevor Weston, M.D.

Contemporary Books, Inc.
Chicago

Library of Congress Cataloging in Publication Data

Weston, Trevor.
  A doctor's guide to home medical care.

  Includes index.
  1. Medicine, Popular.   I. Title.
RC81.W5   1982   616.02'4   81-69607
ISBN 0-8092-5971-0   AACR2

The tables appearing on page 141 are reprinted by permission
of Publications International, Ltd.

Published by Contemporary Books, Inc.
180 North Michigan Avenue, Chicago, Illinois 60601
Manufactured in the United States of America
Library of Congress Catalog Card Number: 81-69607
International Standard Book Number: 0-8092-5971-0

Published simultaneously in Canada by
Beaverbooks, Ltd.
150 Lesmill Road
Don Mills, Ontario M3B 2T5
Canada

Contents

Acknowledgments   vii
Introduction   ix
1/Serious or Not?   1
2/Treating Yourself   5
3/Home Medicine Chest   7
4/First Aid and Emergency Care   13
5/What You Should Do   19
6/Home Nursing Care   107
7/How to Stay Healthy   127
8/Staying on Top   139
9/Avoiding Trouble   183
10/Medical Care   197
Appendix—An Exercise Program   205
Index   223

Acknowledgments

No book of this sort, even if it comes from one pen, can really be the fruit of a single mind and I am conscious that in it I am largely passing on what I have learned from others as well as what I have experienced myself. I am particularly indebted to my colleague Miss Evelyn Brown, Executive Editor of the British Medical Association's Family Doctor Publications unit and to Dr. H. Wykeham Balme, Consultant Physician at St. Bartholomew's Hospital, London, for their invaluable contribution in independently scrutinizing the text, and to Mrs. Carol Young for undertaking the mammoth typing task involved. My grateful thanks are also due to the Health Education Council of Great Britain for permission to reproduce material originally published by them.

My greatest debt, however, is to my patients who in the course of the past twenty-five years have been my real teachers.

Introduction

All of us get worried when things go wrong with our health or when we feel ill. We often tend to think the worst but then do little or nothing because we are afraid—usually quite unconsciously—of learning the truth in case it turns out to be unpleasant. Sometimes even the most strong-minded of us panic and do whatever comes into our heads first. Unfortunately that may be the wrong thing to do. So the purpose of this book is to tell you what to do when things go wrong. The book is intended to be straightforward, down-to-earth, and practical. The book has been written with the belief that even though people's workings and misworkings are complex, they can be presented in ways that not only make them understandable but constitute an exciting voyage of exploration and discovery. It is not, however, a do-it-yourself medical guide: first, because what is presented between these covers is only a fraction of what your doctor needs to know to handle all the situations that may confront him; second, because although most people work and go wrong in broadly similar ways, the art of successful medical management lies in peoples' differences; and third, because book-learning is only a part of what makes up your doctor's skill. The main part of your doctor's skill involves seeing your illness not so much against the background he has obtained from books and lectures but against the experience he has gained from looking after thousands of other people.

We live in a world of surprising contrasts. A world in which many people are more familiar with the structure of the moon and the insides of a computer than with the appearance and function of their own digestive system. A dangerous world, fraught with the hazards of death and injury from a nuclear catastrophe, global pollution, and overpopulation. A world even more fraught with the follies of ignorance and misunderstanding. For ours is a world in which enough is known in the field of medical science for it to make a substantial difference in life or death, health or disease, happiness or suffering. Health care will make a substantial difference, however, only if we know how to use available medical knowledge.

Most of us—no matter how young—are not nearly as likely to be personally injured, let alone killed, by the effects of a nuclear catastrophe, pollution, or overpopulation as we are by disease. Disease is the unsuspected enemy that lurks within us. Three things—all under our control—give that deadly enemy unnecessary advantages. The first is that we give more thought to what is happening to the man on the moon than to what is happening to our own health. We act as if we had ninety lives instead of only one or as if we expected our good health to continue forever. The second is that we do not take steps to avoid or prevent diseases and suffering that are unnecessary and wasteful both to ourselves and to those who care for us. Disease and disability are terrible enough when they are inevitable or unavoidable. When they could have been prevented, they bring on the added tragedy of the life, the talent, and the opportunities that were unnecessarily cut short. The third is that when we become ill, we do not make use of the medical services that are available to us nearly as well as we might. We fail to get as much benefit as we could from what modern medicine can offer.

All too often—and all too tragically—the outcome of illness depends on whether we take full advantage of what modern medicine can do for us. Most of us know less about how our bodies and minds work, what can go wrong with them, and what we can do to keep them healthy than about any other aspect of our lives—even though all other aspects of our lives are dependent on our bodies and minds continuing to work effortlessly and effectively every day and every night. It is my hope that this book will help you and your family to take full, sensible, and early advantage of all the help that your doctor can offer you nowadays.

1.
Serious or Not?

The most important, yet sometimes the most difficult, decision that we must make about an illness is whether or not it is serious. Should you get medical advice about your ailment, or can you safely wait to see what happens or cope with it on your own? If your ailment is serious enough to see your doctor about, how soon should you see him? Can you wait until office hours tomorrow or even for an appointment next week, or should you ask your doctor to see you at once? About obvious emergencies on the one hand and trivial conditions on the other, there is seldom much doubt. Difficulties arise when an illness could be serious or not. The seriousness of a disease depends on several considerations, but nearly all are related to the nature of the symptoms.

The symptoms of an illness are what you, the patient, notice to be out of the ordinary and feel to be wrong with you; the signs of the illness are what your doctor finds wrong with you when he examines you. There are two broad groups of symptoms: those that appear in the particular part of the body that is disordered—such as the sore throat in tonsillitis—

which are called local symptoms, and those that affect your body as a whole—such as a vague feeling of illness—which are regarded as general symptoms. Local symptoms usually include pain, inflammation, swelling, a lump, a blemish, or a discharge. General symptoms may include malaise, lethargy or lassitude, loss of appetite (anorexia) or weight, raised temperature or fever, or a rash.

Whenever you are ill, the first step is to make note of your symptoms and classify them as local or general. The next step is to assess their severity. The assessment of the severity of symptoms is difficult because symptoms are subjective; they cannot be compared to objective standards or measurements. Almost literally, an overall feeling of illness that one man will shrug off will keep another away from work for a week, and one man's agony will be as slight as a pinprick to another. Nevertheless, after accounting for the related factors of personality, thresholds and tolerances for pain and illness, and any possible secondary gains to be made by declaring or concealing illness, we must come to a conclusion about the significance of our symptoms.

We think of severe symptoms as indications of serious disorders and slight symptoms as indications of minor illnesses, and we generally are right. Sometimes, however, we unconsciously deceive ourselves and incorrectly evaluate our symptoms. Symptoms that involve unpleasantness or discomfort, such as pain or vomiting, and those that lead to incapacity or disability and interfere with work or play usually are correctly interpreted as potentially serious. We may be even more concerned and more ready to seek advice about symptoms that are minor but that cause shame or embarrassment, such as spots or smells, or symptoms that worry us because we think they may be due to something serious, such as heart disease or cancer. Some people delay or even refuse to seek medical advice because they are afraid—often quite mistakenly—that their symptoms must be due to a serious or incurable condition which they would rather not know about. They will suffer, whatever the real answer proves to be. They will alarm themselves, and often spend sleepness nights, un-necessarily, if they have a minor disease. And they will lose the chance for curative treatment if they have a major problem.

But what are we to do? On the one hand, we are constantly reminded that delay in consulting a doctor can be dangerous and can mean loss of the chance of a cure of a serious illness. On the other, we do not want to trouble the doctor needlessly, make a fuss about something that turns out to be trivial, or risk getting the reputation of being a hypochondriac. Here are some guidelines:

If something is going wrong, unless you are sure that you know what it is and can handle it yourself, see your doctor about it as soon as you can get an appointment. Never delay for more than a few days; to do so will certainly cost you peace of mind and maybe much more. Still it is worthwhile to get a sense of priorities and time frames. Your doctor is as interested in quickly treating your illness and relieving your anxiety as you are. And he will be pleased to be able to tell you that your symptoms are not due to anything serious. He won't regard finding out that nothing much is wrong as a waste of his time; he knows only too well that the early symptoms of disease may be slight and that early diagnosis often makes all the difference to an eventually successful outcome. He always will be saddened to discover that because of unnecessary delay somebody has passed a sentence of death on himself. But he is equally likely to be angry if he is called out at night or on a weekend to deal with something that has been going on for days or even weeks. Although there are exceptions, serious symptoms that come on quickly, or rapidly get worse, need prompt attention; symptoms that are not serious but prevent sleep or keep you in bed call for attention the next day. Other conditions should be dealt with as soon as possible, both to relieve your anxiety about them and to get the benefit of early diagnosis and treatment. But don't try to diagnose serious or persistent symptoms. Diagnosing a problem may appear to be easy and may even be self-evident, but it often is the most difficult aspect of managing an illness—even for a doctor. It is also the most important aspect; deciding on the proper treatment and the eventual outcome of the disease depends upon it. It's much too serious a matter to take chances with; leave it to an expert. Finally, if you are in doubt about whether or not to go to your doctor, go!

2.

Treating Yourself

If you decide that there is nothing seriously wrong with you and that you can deal with the problem yourself without medical advice, how much and what can you safely do? In the pages that follow, we shall consider the evaluation and treatment of common symptoms and emergencies individually, in alphabetical order, and suggest what you can reasonably and safely do to help yourself. Certainly you can treat many minor illnesses and accidents without bothering your doctor. But be sure not to tackle any illness unless you are sure that it is minor and that you know what you are trying to achieve with your home treatment. (Details of particular kinds of care and nursing at home are found on pages 107–25.) Over-the-counter drugs play a definite and useful part in the management of minor illnesses, but they also pose possible dangers. Take care to follow the instructions on the bottle, and don't take twice as much as recommended in the hope of getting a quick result. And never, ever, take medicine out of a bottle that has lost its label. Don't continue taking drugs on your own for too long without seeking help. If there is no improvement within two days at the most, you definitely should see your doctor. People who take over-the-counter medicines for weeks on end for indigestion or a cough are asking for serious trouble; the damage inside may be steadily getting worse while people continue with improper treatment.

If you have been taking medicine on your own for some time before seeing your doctor, make sure that you tell him about it; the drugs may have altered the pattern of your illness. Remember, too, that most over-the-counter drugs work not by curing the disease but by relieving the symptoms until the body puts things right again. You may be deluded into thinking that the medicine must have cured the condition because the symptoms went away and that all you need do is take the medicine every time the symptoms recur. If symptoms come back at all, you probably have something that your body can't cure on its own. The sensible thing to do then is not to take any more medicine—even though it is a quick and easy answer—but to get the condition properly investigated.

Help from the pharmacist. A great deal of advice about caring for minor illnesses and choosing home remedies can be obtained from a pharmacist. Remember that the pharmacist has undergone comprehensive training, and his knowledge of what can go wrong with you and how medicine can make it right is second only to the doctor's. Although his business is selling medicines to the public as well as preparing doctors' prescriptions, the pharmacist works under a strict code of professional conduct. He can be relied upon to give unbiased advice, and he will not hesitate to refuse to sell medicine to somebody whom he thinks should have medical advice instead. So even though you may purchase drugs from any pharmacist, you will be wise to choose and stick to one. You should form a relationship with the pharmacist so he knows the medicines that you take and your medical background and so he can give you satisfactory advice whenever necessary. The choice of a regular pharmacist is almost as important as the choice of a personal doctor.

3.

Home Medicine Chest

Every home should have a medicine chest that contains simple equipment, dressings, and drugs for use in emergencies and accidents and for treating minor illnesses. All the medicines that any member of the family takes should be kept in the medicine chest. The chest should also have a list of phone numbers that may be needed in an emergency—doctor, hospital, ambulance, etc.—pasted on the inside of the door or lid. It should have an envelope containing cards that list important points about the medical history of each member of the household. The cards should note any previous illnesses and operations, allergies and sensitivities, immunization records, and drugs that must be taken regularly.

Mark the medicine chest clearly, and make sure that everybody in the family knows where it is. Don't keep medicines anywhere else in the house, and keep the medicine cabinet out of the reach of small children. Many medicines look temptingly like sweets, and poisoning is one of the most common causes of accidental death of children. Check the contents of the cabinet regularly and replace items as they are used. Take back to the pharmacist or flush down the toilet (do not discard drugs in the garbage) all unlabeled and expired medicines.

Before taking any medicine, check the label on the bottle. Never take more or less than is recommended without consulting your doctor. Take care to follow any other directions about the frequency or the time of the day to take the drugs.

The well-stocked medicine cabinet includes:

Equipment

Safety pins (medium and large)
Scissors (5″ blunt ended, stainless steel)
Tweezers (blunt ended)

Thermometer
Flashlight (with spare battery and bulb)
Pad and pencil

Medicine measuring cup
Dropper (for eye, ear, or nose drops)

Dressings

Wound dressings (small, medium, and large)
Sterile bandage rolls (1″, 2″, and 3″)
Elastic bandages (2″ and 3″)

Triangular bandages for use as slings
Gauze
Cotton balls

Adhesive tape (1″ wide)

Adhesive strips (2½″ wide)
Adhesive bandages (assorted sizes)
Eye pad (sterilized, with bandage)

Medicines

Aspirin or acetaminophen (as found in Tylenol) tablets for pain or fever
Antacid tablets for indigestion
Antidiarrhea mixture
Two types of cough medicine—a suppressant to relieve a dry cough and an

expectorant to help get up sputum from a wet cough
Children's aspirin, antidiarrhea, and cough mixtures
Antiseptic solution or cream
Calamine lotion or cream for itchy rashes, bites, and sunburn

Zinc oxide ointment and castor oil cream for sore areas
Liniment for massaging sore muscles
Gargle and mild lozenges for a sore throat
Inhalants (menthol or eucalyptus) for a cough or hoarseness

MAKING THE MOST OF THE MEDICINE
IN YOUR MEDICINE CHEST

Keep your nonprescription drugs few and simple, and get to know them well. If necessary, ask your pharmacist to help you.

Aspirin (acetylsalicylic acid) or acetaminophen (as found in Tylenol and other non-aspirin brands). Aspirin and acetaminophen have a similar action and are equally effective, but many people find that one suits them better than the other. Decide which you prefer and stock it; don't keep both on hand. If you do choose aspirin, remember to dissolve the tablets in at least a cup of water; the drug will irritate your stomach less. If you have ever had a peptic ulcer, frequently have indigestion, or take anticoagulant tablets, avoid aspirin completely.

Remember that aspirin and acetaminophen don't cure anything; they merely help relieve pain and fever. If you need to take either drug for more than two or three days, you probably have an illness that will not go away by itself, and you should see your doctor about it. The usual dosage for aspirin or acetaminophen is two tablets every four hours up to a maximum of twelve a day. Both types of tablets maintain their strength and are safe to use for at least two years if kept in a tightly closed bottle away from any dampness.

Antacids. When taking an antacid, suck or chew the tablets; don't swallow them. If you find antacid tablets are unpleasant because they are too gritty, ask your pharmacist about the alternatives. A liquid antacid often works better and more quickly than tablets, but it is inconvenient to carry around. Antacid tablets can be taken as often as necessary; two 5 ml (1 teaspoon) doses of the liquid may be taken about an hour after each meal up to four times a day.

Antidiarrhea mixture. A common antidiarrhea agent is kaolin (as found in such over-the-counter brands as Donnegal, Kaopectate, and Parapectolin). It may be taken in a dose of 20 ml at first and then in two 5 ml doses every three hours until diarrhea improves. Kaolin should be stopped as soon as the bowels are back to normal, or you may become constipated instead. If you still have diarrhea after two days, it's time to see your doctor.

Cough medicines. Coughing is nature's way of clearing undesirable material out of the lungs and therefore should be encouraged. Nevertheless, use of a cough medicine is sometimes reasonable (see page 42 for details). If a cough persists for more than a week, consult your doctor.

Children's medicines. Children may receive aspirin, acetaminophen, kaolin, or a cough suppressant in the following doses:

Up to one year, give a basic dose of 5 ml (1 teaspoon).
One to five years, give two basic doses.
Five to eight years, give three basic doses.
Eight to twelve years, give four basic doses.
Over twelve years, give the adult dose.

Aspirin or acetaminophen may be given every four to six hours; kaolin every four hours.

Children who have a dry cough that interferes with sleep may receive a cough suppressant a half-hour before going to bed and again if the child is awakened by the cough during the night.

Antiseptics. There are many effective antiseptic solutions and creams on the market.

Skin preparation. Your skin is highly sensitive tissue; so take care what you put on it. We suggest only three preparations for your medicine chest—calamine lotion, zinc oxide, or castor oil cream. If any of these is not effective, see your doctor.

Throat preparations. Both gargles and lozenges can help relieve a sore throat (see page 91). Hot salt water or aspirin gargles (two teaspoons of salt or two aspirin tablets dissolved in a cup of hot water) are as good as any. The aspirin solution should be swallowed after gargling so it can do some good internally as well. For lozenges, one fruit troche sucked slowly per hour is satisfactory.

Inhalants. Add one teaspoon of a menthol and eucalyptus

inhalant mixture to two cups of hot—but not boiling—water in a basin or jug. Drape a towel over your head and round the basin or jug to form a tent. With your mouth open, take long slow breaths.

Laxative. Laxatives have no place in a sensible home, and their use should be avoided. The management of constipation is discussed on pages 38–40.

Eye preparations. Sore eyes may be helped by bathing them with warm salt water. A pinch of salt in an inch of warm boiled water in an eyecup may be held over the open eye a half-dozen times for ten seconds each time. If there is no improvement the next day, see your doctor.

Eye drops or ointments should not be used unless they have been ordered by your doctor. To place drops in the eye, separate the eyelids using the finger and thumb of one hand. With the other hand, squeeze out the drops onto the outer edge of the eye so they run across the eye. Two or three drops usually are sufficient.

Ear preparations. Warm olive oil may be used to soften wax, but then only if you are sure that your eardrums are not perforated. Otherwise, do not put drops into your ears unless ordered by your doctor. To put drops in the ear, lie down or hold your head to one side and place three or four drops into the ear. Remain in that position for five to ten minutes so that the drops have time to do their work.

Nose preparations. Drops containing ephedrine may relieve a running nose. Ephedrine is an alkaloid derived from leaves of *ephedra equisetina* and acts to dilate the bronchial tubes. It is found in Chlor-Trimeton and other brands of nasal drops (be sure to read the label for ingredients). When taking them, tip your head as far back as you can and insert four drops slowly into each side of the nose. If the drops run down onto your lip, or you feel them running down the back of your throat, your head isn't tilted back far enough. *Do not* use a nasal spray or drops more than four times a day or for more than four days. Prolonged use of nose drops will damage the lining of the nose and cause chronic nasal inflammation.

4.

First Aid
and
Emergency Care

Sooner or later, many of us will encounter an accident or medical emergency. How we react and what we do can make a substantial difference in the outcome.

FIRST AID PLAN

The purpose of first aid is to keep the victim's condition from getting worse by giving essential emergency treatment—but no more than that—and obtaining medical aid. Try to work out carefully what you are going to do, rather than doing the first thing that comes to mind. Remember that, apart from organizing medical help, often the best thing to do is nothing. The temptation to do something can be not only dangerous but almost overwhelming. Remember, too, that heroic measures are almost always harmful. If in doubt, do nothing!

Doing things in the right order is very important:

1. *Avoid further injury.* Try to drag the victim away from the scene of the accident and out of range of further injury.

You may need to establish traffic control before you can attend to the victim. And you must take care that you don't become a casualty yourself.

2. *Help your victim to breathe.* Look for movement of the chest or abdomen or listen at the mouth or nose for signs of breathing. If there is none, search the mouth for any obstruction, such as dentures, vomit, or blood, and remove it. Then place the head as far back as possible and begin resuscitation (see pages 31–34).

3. *Stop severe bleeding.* Apply firm and persistent pressure with the flat of your hand, your fist, or a pad directly on the wound. If a limb is injured, hold it upright to help control bleeding (see pages 25–29).

4. *Carefully position unconscious victims.* Make sure that an unconscious accident victim is lying on his belly with his head to one side and tipped back in the "recovery position" (see page 98). If possible, position the victim so his body is tilted and his head is lower than his feet.

5. *Cover any serious wounds or burns with a clean handkerchief or scarf.*

6. *Prevent movement of any part of the body that looks as though it is the site of a fracture; if possible, immobilize it.*

7. *Get help.* Get too much rather than too little help. Give information about the location of the accident and the number of victims and nature of the injuries as precisely as you can.

8. *Give tender loving care.* A victim will be shocked and frightened; so reassure and comfort him. Cover him, with your own coat if necessary, but with only one layer of clothing on top of his own clothes. Do not, even if he begs you, give the victim anything to eat or drink. Food or liquid may seriously interfere with a subsequent anesthetic or aggravate internal injuries. If the victim has been burned, you should, however, give him water to replace the fluid he is losing (see page 37).

The order in which you take these actions may vary according to the circumstances of the particular accident. But do make sure that you get the priorities of first aid in the right order It would be tragic if somebody choked on his false teeth while you were attending to a relatively harmless wound on his leg.

ACCIDENT PLAN

If you come across an auto crash, take these steps:

1. Position your car, off the road if possible, so your headlights will give maximum illumination of the scene of the accident and switch on your warning lights.

2. Organize traffic control. Place red, flashing warning lights if you have them 200 yards from the accident in both directions. Make sure that you don't become a casualty yourself.

3. Put out any fire. Use an extinguisher or smother the flames with earth.

4. Switch off the ignition and lights of the wrecked car and apply the handbrake.

5. Check all victims before getting to work on any one of them. Ask any conscious victims how many people were in the vehicle. Quickly look behind hedges or other obstructions for people who may have been thrown by the impact. Harden your heart to the cries of those in great pain and your natural inclination to linger with the dead. The unconscious have the greatest need of your attention.

6. Begin giving first aid as described on the previous page. Apart from getting them out of the way of further danger and putting them in the "recovery position," move victims as little as possible. The danger of compounding their injuries is considerable. Only move victims if absolutely essential—do so only to protect them from the danger of further injury.

7. Get the next person to arrive at the scene of the accident to inform the ambulance and police services, giving the location, the number of victims, and the nature of the injuries as precisely as possible. Second and third helpers

should be asked to attend to traffic and crowd control. You and any subsequent first-aid workers need the entire accident area to work in, clear of the panic, advice, or interference of onlookers. Remember that all your efforts will come to naught if blocked roads prevent ambulances and other rescue vehicles from getting to the casualties.

FIRE PLAN

In case of fire, follow an organized plan. First, do not rush into a burning building without stopping to think, or you may become the only fatality. Ask yourself if it is likely that someone is inside. If so, ask yourself if there is a reasonable chance that the person is still alive and that you will be able to get him and yourself out before the fire engulfs the building or the floors collapse. If you can see somebody inside, decide whether he is trapped and needs your assistance or whether you would do better to direct his efforts to escape from outside.

If you do go inside a burning building, remember that smoke kills far more people by asphyxiation than flames do by burning. A wet handkerchief placed over your mouth and nose will give you some protection. Smoke rises, even in a closed room, so stay low. If necessary, move on your hands and knees. Be very cautions about opening doors so you don't get caught in a wall of flame. When you get to a victim, proceed as on pages 13–14.

1. If the fire is in your own home or office: do what you can to put it out. Use an extinguisher or a fire blanket if there is one; otherwise use water, sand, or earth. *Never* throw water on a frying pan or electrical fire; use sand or earth or try to smother flames with a rug, towel, or blanket. *Never* try to carry a blazing frying pan to the sink or anywhere else. The pan probably will burn your hand, and the flames will flare up in your face.

2. Close all the doors and windows to reduce drafts.

3. Check that all electricity in the burning room is switched off, and, as soon as possible, switch off electricity in the whole house.

4. Call the fire department yourself. Do not assume that someone else has.

5. Warn everybody in the building and make sure that they leave it. If possible, have a roll call outside.

6. If you are trapped in the building, make the room as airtight as possible by closing the door and the windows and trying to block gaps under doors, etc. If the room is full of smoke, lie on the floor. The air often is fresh there. Breathe slowly and deliberately, trying not to panic. If the smoke becomes suffocating, hold your breath, dash for the window, and lean as far out as you can. Never jump unless there is absolutely no alternative and you face certain death. If there is no prospect of rescue in time and you have the facilities, knot together sheets, blankets, or curtains, to make a rope. Make sure that the rope is securely anchored. If you can, throw bedding or cushions onto the ground where you expect to land. Lower yourself out of the window slowly, feet first, and try to land with your knees bent.

7. Deal with clothing or victims on fire, and burns, as detailed on pages 13–14, and 37.

5.

What You Should Do

The purpose of this chapter is to give you advice about what to do when you are faced with a common medical problem or emergency. The section indicates how urgent a problem is by telling you when to see your doctor. It presents degrees of urgency as follows:

Now—the circumstances about which you should see your doctor or get to the nearest hospital, by ambulance if necessary.

Within 12 hours—the circumstances about which you should see your doctor.

Within 24 hours—the circumstances about which you should see your doctor.

Within 7 days—the circumstances about which you should see your doctor.

BUT IF YOU ARE IN DOUBT ABOUT THE URGENCY OF A MEDICAL PROBLEM, PHONE AND ASK TO SEE YOUR DOCTOR AT ONCE.

This chapter also includes suggestions about the course of action that you should follow and, where appropriate, presents information about:

What your doctor may do. These paragraphs are intended to give you some idea of what to expect. Your doctor is not a technician who goes through a set routine of examination procedures and special tests. He is a unique mixture of scientist, artist, and magician whose training and experience have taught him that although "cases" have much in common, no two are alike. Consequently what he feels is necessary to arrive at a conclusion about your particular case may not follow a standard pattern.

What you can do. These paragraphs present reliable and safe measures that you can take to resolve the medical problem or to be of help until you see your doctor.

ACHING

see PAIN, page 76

ANAL

Bleeding—commonly due to hemorrhoids, an external or internal crack or tear (fissure), inflammation of the colon (colitis or dysentery), or a growth in the colon or rectum.

Discharge—commonly due to inflammation of the rectum (proctitis) or possibly due to gonorrhea.

Itching (pruritus)—commonly due to hemorrhoids, a fissure, diarrhea, soiling, discharge, worms, eczema, or stress.

Lumps—commonly due to hemorrhoids, warts, protrusion (prolapse) of the rectum.

Pain—commonly due to hemorrhoids (especially if they are inflammed or clotted), rectal spasm (proctalgia fugax), a fissure, an abscess, an abnormal opening (fistula), or cancer.

You Should See Your Doctor about an Anal Problem:

If *any* of these symptoms persists for more than five days or returns within six months.

What your doctor may do. Your doctor may examine the

skin around the anus and the inside of anus with a gloved finger or a small metal instrument (proctoscope) that has been lubricated to minimize discomfort. In some cases, an X-ray of the lower bowel (barium enema) or a more extensive examination (sigmoidoscopy) may be necessary. Laboratory tests on the stools also may be necessary.

What you can do. Avoid scratching. Avoid constipation; if necessary take a laxative, but only for a few days. Take extra care about keeping the area clean; wash it after each bowel movement. Pain can be eased by placing on the anus a flannel cloth that has been soaked in hot or very cold water. Itching can be reduced by applying zinc oxide or castor oil cream. Suppositories are sometimes helpful, but they should not be used without consulting your doctor or pharmacist.

ANXIETY

see EMOTIONAL AND MENTAL DISORDERS, page 51 and pages 158–67

APPETITE

Too little (anorexia)—may be due to a digestive upset, an infectious disease (especially an intestinal infection), cancer (particularly of the digestive tract), emotional disorders (especially anorexia nervosa), chronic liver or kidney disorders, or conditions that interfere with taste or smell (for example, the common cold).

Changes in appetite are difficult to assess accurately, but they inevitably are followed by a corresponding change in weight. If you suspect your appetite has decreased substantially, check your weight once a week on the same scale in similar clothes and at the same time of day. Most often, a loss of appetite is temporary. Persistent anorexia and weight loss, however, can be early indications of serious disease and should not be allowed to continue for more than a few weeks without consulting your doctor. In the meantime, you may try to stimulate your appetite by taking an *aperitif* a half-hour before you plan to eat.

Too much—can be due to habitual overeating, diabetes, an overactive thyroid gland (people who have diabetes or an overactive thyroid usually lose weight despite the extra food they eat), loneliness and depression ("consolation" eating), or intestinal worms (a doubtful but traditional cause).

The appetite is normally increased, but nevertheless should be watched, in growing children, pregnant women, and individuals who are strenuously exercising. (The dangers of being overweight and what you should do about it are presented on pages 140–54.) You should take steps, with your doctor's help if necessary, as soon as your weight begins to creep up. The higher you let it go before doing something, the more difficult weight loss will be.

BITES AND STINGS

Animal—The danger from animal bites is due to organisms on the animal's tongue or in its saliva that get into your body through the wound. The chance of a serious problem resulting from an animal bite is small. However, since you cannot be sure which animals carry dangerous organisms and which do not, you should take precautions in all cases, and the sooner the better.

You Should See Your Doctor about a Bite:

Now If the animal was rabid, if the wounds are extensive, or if you are frightened or shocked.

Within 24 hours If you have never had a complete course of three antitetanus injections, or you have not had a booster injection within the last five years; if the area around the wound becomes tender, red, or swollen; or if you develop a fever.

What your doctor may do. Your doctor will clean and sterilize the wound and assess the need for stitches. He will assess the need for antirabies treatment and give an antitetanus injection if necessary. He also will determine the need for prescribing an antibiotic.

What you can do. Hold the wound under running water, then soak it in warm water before cleaning it thoroughly with soap or an antiseptic. Apply antiseptic lotion or cream. Cover the wound if the bite is on a part of the body that is exposed to dirt. Repeat the procedure three times a day until the wound begins to heal.

Insect—Swelling and pain at the site of the sting, especially from bees or horseflies, may be greater than you expect, and they may last for several hours. The only real danger is if you are allergic to venom, in which case you will go into shock or collapse and obviously need help.

You Should See Your Doctor about the Sting:

Now If you start going into shock, feel faint, or collapse; if in the past you had an intense reaction to an insect bite or sting, involving fainting, difficult breathing, or a generalized rash.

Within 24 hours If the swelling or pain persist (possibly due to infection in the wound).

What your doctor may do. Your doctor will treat shock, difficult breathing, or rash, depending on the severity, by giving an injection of adrenalin or antihistamine tablets or injection. Hospital treatment usually is necessary only for care of a severe reaction.

What you can do. Give first aid for shock, if necessary, as described on page 89. Then remove the sting. Grasp the insect's sting as close to the skin surface as possible to avoid squeezing more venom into your body. Remove the sting with tweezers or scrubbed fingers by pulling or scraping against the direction of entry. Bathe the wound with disinfectant. Apply ice or a cold compress as quickly as possible to minimize the local reaction. Later, if irritation and pain are bothersome, apply a soothing lotion (such as calamine) or cream (such as zinc oxide or castor oil) and take aspirin or acetaminophen. Avoid scratching, which may cause infection of the wound. Rest the affected part by placing the arm in a sling or putting the leg up on a chair.

Snake—Most snake bites occur on the lower leg or hand. If you are traveling in snake-infested country, take care where you put your hands and feet, and wear boots or leggings and gloves.

You Should See a Doctor about the Bite:

Now If you think there is any likelihood that the snake was venomous. Kill the snake and take it with you or memorize a description of it so it can be identified later. If the snake probably was venomous, begin first aid measures immediately and ask the doctor to come to you.

What the doctor may do. The doctor probably will give an injection of the appropriate antivenom and deal with the wound and shock as necessary.

What you can do. If the snake was venomous, act quickly and decisively. Lie down and keep the affected part still; movement increases the spread of the poison. Immediately apply a tourniquet to obstruct the veins. Tie a handkerchief, necktie, or scarf directly above the bite to stop the poison from spreading to the rest of the body. If the hand or foot becomes blue, loosen the tourniquet every fifteen minutes for about a minute. If you have a sharp knife or razor blade, make incisions on the fang marks at 45-degree angles and suck out the venom. At least half the poison can be eliminated in this way if performed within 15 minutes of the bite. If possible, sterilize the blade before using it. The cuts should be about a quarter-inch long and not more than a quarter-inch deep. If you spit out the poison and rinse your mouth afterward, there is little chance you will be affected by the venom. Splint the limb as if it were fractured before moving to the hospital.

BLEEDING

From wounds—Light bleeding usually stops quickly and does not require treatment other than care of the wound. When large amounts of blood are lost quickly (hemorrhage), urgent effective action is necessary to save life. The primary tasks are to control the bleeding and minimize the effects of shock (see SHOCK, pages 88–90).

What you can do. First, remove any foreign body—shell, splinter, glass, clothing, etc.—that can easily be picked out of the wound. If possible, grasp the wound firmly between your thumb and fingers so that you pull the edge and the underlying tissues together and then hold them pressed against each other. At the same time push down on the wound. In this way, you control bleeding from the blood vessels near the surface of the skin and from those lying more deeply. You may first have to tear away clothing to get to the wound. If the wound is large, gaping, or open, watch where the blood is spurting from. Push your clenched fist onto that area. Don't worry about dirty hands. Your patient would rather be alive with an infected wound than dead with a clean one.

You must keep pressing the edges of the wound together and pushing down on the site of bleeding until a pressure dressing is applied or until the bleeding stops. If a large artery has been cut, bleeding may continue for quite some time. To avoid undoing the good you have done by releasing the pressure too soon and allowing the hemorrhage to recur, try to keep applying pressure for ten minutes (by the clock); then slacken the pressure gradually so you can immediately increase it if necessary. In the meantime, try to get your patient to sit or lie down, and, unless you suspect a fracture, try to raise the bleeding part to decrease the flow of blood.

As soon as you can, apply a pressure dressing to the wound.

The dressing must be heavy, thick, and large enough to extend well beyond the edges of the wound. A tightly folded cloth or a rolled up bandage may be used. If the wound is gaping, the dressing must be packed into it and not just stretched across the top of it. Do not slacken pressure on the wound until the dressing is in place and has been firmly fixed in position by adhesive.

If blood begins to soak through the dressing, don't remove the dressing, add more padding and bandage the wound more firmly. Consider applying a tourniquet only if blood is soaking through the dressings faster than you can control or if the wound is too big for you to exert pressure with your hands. If you must use a tourniquet, place it between the wound and the trunk and tighten it just enough to control the bleeding; remember to release the tourniquet for a few seconds every ten minutes to avoid seriously damaging the limb.

Finally, immobilize the injured part of the body, guard against shock, and arrange for medical care.

From the ear—Bleeding from the ear is most commonly due to a tear in the ear's lining after somebody has tried to remove wax with a matchstick or a hairpin. It can be due to more serious causes, such as a rupture of the eardrum as the result of injury or infection or a fracture of the base of the skull.

You Should See Your Doctor about Bleeding from Inside the Ear:

Now If there has been a recent blow or injury to the head.

Within 12 hours If there is also pain, discharge, deafness, or pronounced giddiness.

Within 24 hours In all other cases, to make sure that bleeding was not due to anything serious.

What your doctor may do. Your doctor will look inside your ear with a special instrument (otoscope) or a head mirror to find out the location of the bleeding. If necessary, he may order an X-ray of the skull or refer you to an ear specialist.

What you can do. Do not put in ear drops or a plug of cotton. If bleeding from the ear follows an injury to the head, lay the patient on his side with the affected ear turned down.

From the nose (epistaxis)—Because the blood vessels of the dividing part of the nose (septum) lie close to the surface, they can be damaged and bleed after slight injuries, such as after heavy blowing. A cold or other nasal inflammation makes them even more liable to bleed. Repeated bleeding from the nose in an adult may be due to some general condition, such as high blood pressure or a blood disease. Although the bleeding may appear to be heavy, it rarely is dangerous. Almost all nosebleeds can be stopped at home if you are patient.

You Should See Your Doctor about Bleeding from the Nose:

> **Now** If it has persisted for twenty minutes or follows a recent blow or injury to the head.

Within 7 days If it happens repeatedly.

What your doctor may do. The doctor will look inside your nose with a special instrument (nasal speculum) to identify the source of the bleeding. He possibly will pack the nose with gauze. He also will check for high blood pressure and bleeding disorders. If necessary, he will send you to the hospital so the problem can be corrected by cauterization.

What you can do. Sit down with your head bent slightly forward over a bowl. Pinch the lower, soft part of your nose between a finger and thumb for at least five minutes (by the clock). You can spit out any blood that gets into your throat, but do not blow your nose for at least a half-hour. Then blow gently so you don't start the nose bleeding again.

In the mouth—Bleeding from the mouth is commonly due to injury to the lips, gums, or tongue; unhealed sockets after teeth have been removed; inflamed gums (gingivitis); and blood dripping down from the back of the nose. It also can be due to more serious problems in the stomach or lungs.

Blood from the stomach may be vomited. It may be mixed with recently eaten, partly digested food and look like coffee grounds. Blood from the lungs may be coughed up and may be frothy or rust colored. Strenuous coughing, for any reason, may produce blood-streaked phlegm. Be sure to get your doctor's opinion about bloody phlegm, especially if it occurs repeatedly.

You Should See Your Doctor about Bleeding in the Mouth:

Now If blood is repeatedly vomited in the course of an hour or if the total quantity is more than a pint; if it is coughed up repeatedly in the course of an hour or if the total quantity is more than an eggcup full; if there is persistent bleeding from the tongue, lips, gums, or a tooth socket for more than an hour.

Within 12 hours In all other cases of vomiting blood or "coffee grounds," coughing up blood, or having blood-streaked or rust-colored phlegm or spittle.

What your doctor may do. Your doctor will look inside your mouth to see if the source of the bleeding is there. If blood is coming from a wound in the lip, tongue, or gums, he may stitch it. If blood comes from a tooth socket, he may pack the socket with a dental dressing. If your symptoms indicate that the blood is coming from your stomach or lungs, your doctor may arrange for you to be admitted to a hospital for further investigation of the cause and appropriate treatment.

What you can do. If the cause of the bleeding is obvious (for instance, a tooth socket), you may be able to control it by biting firmly on a bandage roll or other pad that has been placed directly over the bleeding area. Bleeding from cuts on the lips and tongue may be controlled by holding the edges of the wound firmly together between fingers and thumb. If someone has been bleeding heavily from the stomach or lungs, he may be going into shock and require prompt treatment to reverse it (see SHOCK, page 89). Remember not to give him anything to eat or drink.

From the anus or rectum—see ANAL, Bleeding, pages 20–21
In the urine—see URINARY CONDITIONS, page 99
From the vagina—Normal causes of bleeding from the vagina are menstruation and recent childbirth. Common abnormal causes are irregular menstrual cycles, threatened miscarriage, inflammation of the genital tract, fibroids or tumors of the womb (uterus). The bleeding may come from the vagina itself, but much more commonly it comes from the uterus. Bleeding from the urethra or anus sometimes is mistaken for vaginal bleeding.

You Should See Your Doctor about Vaginal Bleeding:

Now If it is heavy and continuous, especially if you know or suspect that you may be pregnant.

Within 12 hours If it is not heavy, but you know or suspect that you may be pregnant; if it is accompanied by pain in the lower abdomen or fever.

Within 7 days In all other cases. It is particularly important that unexpected bleeding from the vagina, no matter how slight, is investigated if you are over age 40. Such bleeding may be the first indication of still-curable cancer.

What your doctor may do. The doctor will examine your vagina, using a gloved hand and probably an instrument (speculum) and light. If the bleeding is heavy or likely to be due to a miscarriage, he may arrange for you to be admitted to the hospital immediately.

What you can do. If the bleeding is very heavy or you know or suspect that you may be pregnant, lie down and keep as quiet as possible until the doctor or an ambulance arrives.

BLISTERS

Blisters may be due to a burn or scald or to repeated rubbing from badly fitting shoes.

What You Can Do:

Empty only those blisters that are liable to produce further damage or infection by:

1. Cleaning the surface of the blister with soap and water and applying antiseptic.

2. Sterilizing the point of a large needle by holding it in a flame until it is red hot or by putting it in boiling water for ten minutes. Make sure that the needle does not touch anything else before you use it on the blister.

3. Piercing the blister as close to the normal skin as possible and in two places opposite each other. Piercing the blister will not hurt, since the skin of the blister is "dead."

4. Flattening the blister with a clean cotton ball or gauze to press out the fluid. Do not attempt to remove the skin over the blister.

5. Covering the blister with a dressing and keeping it covered until it has healed.

BOILS

Boils are areas of local inflammation which, when large, are called abscesses.

You Should See Your Doctor about a Boil:

Within 7 days If it persists for more than four days or shows any sign of spreading; if red streaks develop in the area; or if there is any tenderness or swelling in nearby lymph glands. Repeated boils should also be reported to the doctor; they may be an indication of more serious underlying disease, such as diabetes.

What your doctor may do. Your doctor may decide that an antibiotic is necessary in addition to the other measures.

What you can do. The aim of treatment is to heal the boil with or without the formation of pus; to get the pus, if it is present, to discharge through the skin as soon as possible; to prevent the infection from spreading; and to relieve pain. Heat applied directly to a boil will help speed up the inflammatory reaction and "burst" the boil to discharge pus. Heat may be applied by using a cloth that has been in boiling water or a kaolin poultice. (A kaolin poultice is made by heating a container of kaolin in a saucepan of boiling water, then spreading the substance on a piece of gauze.) Whichever is used, be sure that the material is not too hot and will not burn the skin. After testing the heat on your own arm, lay the cloth or poultice on the boil and cover it with a cotton ball and a bandage.

Aspirin or acetaminophen may be taken for the pain. Resting the affected part will help promote healing and minimize the pain and the danger of spreading infection. Do not squeeze a boil because it will likely spread the infection.

BREATHING

Stopped (asphyxia, choking, suffocation)—An obstruction to the nose, mouth, throat, or windpipe (trachea) may prevent air from getting to the lungs. If this happens, or if breathing ceases for some other reason, the heart will stop beating in three or four minutes. There is, therefore, a need to act quickly and decisively.

Mouth-to-Mouth Resuscitation

1. Remove the obstruction, which may be obvious (a cord around the neck, a polyethylene bag over the head, a fall of earth in which the patient is buried) or not (food or false teeth blocking the air passages). For less-obvious obstructions, quickly run your fingers around the inside of the mouth and

the back of the throat to make sure you have removed the entire blockage.

2. If someone is choking on something you can't get at with your fingers, he will make a whistling sound as he struggles to breathe. Try to dislodge the obstruction by giving several hard slaps on the back between the shoulder blades, if possible with the body held so the head is tipped downward. A child should be held upside down by his ankles or bent across your thigh with his head hanging down.

3. Sudden, total obstruction of the airway, such as when a piece of food "goes down the wrong way," may have to be dealt with differently. If the patient is sitting or standing, put your arms around him from behind, make a fist with the thumb pointed upward, and place it in the cavity below the lower end of the breastbone. Put the other hand over it and with the full force of both arms thrust upward under the breastbone and ribs. If the patient is on his back, kneel astride him, put the heel of one hand under the breastbone and the heel of the other hand across the back of the first. Then push sharply and forcefully up under the breastbone. This movement is called the *abdominal thrust,* and its aim is to achieve a "pop-gun effect" that will force out the obstruction.

4. If the patient is not breathing in spite of these maneuvers, immediately start mouth-to-mouth resuscitation.

5. Lay the patient on his back on a hard surface (a mattress will not do). Tilt his head as far back as possible. Press the forehead down with the heel of one hand and pinch the nostrils shut with the finger and thumb of that hand. With the other hand, lift the chin up and pull the mouth open.

6. Take a deep breath and, keeping your mouth wide open, seal your lips firmly around the patient's open mouth and blow air into it slowly and steadily until you have none left. The patient's chest should slowly rise as you blow air into his lungs. Alternatively you may breathe into the patient's nose while keeping his mouth closed. With children, place your lips around both mouth and nose.

7. Remove your mouth and watch the patient's chest fall as

the air comes out. Take another deep breath and repeat maneuver 6. Give the first four breaths in quick succession to rapidly replenish the patient's oxygen supply. Then blow in each new breath as soon as the chest falls at a rate of about fourteen times a minute. If the patient vomits, quickly turn his head sideways and scoop the vomit out of his mouth with your finger before giving him another breath.

If the patient's heart has stopped beating, you will see a gradually darkening blue-gray tinge spread over the skin (cyanosis), no pulsation in the carotid artery of the neck, and widely dilated pupils. Strike the chest sharply on the left side of the lower part of the breastbone with the side of your clenched fist. Do this rhythmically for ten seconds, feeling with your other hand for a return of the pulse in the neck.

Cardiac Compression. If this does not happen, you will have to start external cardiac compression. Ideally cardiac compression should be given by a second person while you continue with mouth-to-mouth resuscitation. If you are on your own, you should inflate the lungs once for every five compressions of the heart. If there are two of you, do not act simultaneously but keep the same ratio of one breath to every five compressions.

1. Kneel beside or astride the patient, facing his head. Put the heel of one hand on the lower part of the breastbone and the heel of the other hand across the back of the first.

2. Keeping your arms stiff, rock forward and press firmly down on the breastbone about two inches. Repeat this process at a rate of sixty thrusts a minute for adults (eighty for children, using one hand only, and one hundred thrusts a minute for babies, using only two fingers). Success is indicated by improvement of the skin color, return of the neck pulse, and constriction of the pupils.

Holger-Nielsen Method

Another type of artificial respiration that may be used if the mouth-to-mouth method is not possible because the face has been damaged or the jaw smashed is the Holger-Nielsen Method:

1. Place the patient facedown, arms raised over his head. Bend his elbows and move his head down and to one side and rest it on his hands. Kneel on one knee in front of the patient, facing his head, and place the palm of each hand over the bottom of one of the patient's shoulder blades.

2. Keeping your arms stiff, rock forward and press steadily on the patient with the weight of your body for a count of three.

3. Release the pressure, rock backward, and slide your hands along the patient's arms to grasp them at a point just above the elbows.

4. Complete your backward rock, lifting the patient's elbows off the ground and back with you until you feel resistance at the patient's shoulders.

5. Drop the elbows and begin the cycle again. Repeat it about twelve times a minute.

Silvester Method

A third type of artificial respiration that is particularly useful in cases of facial injury is the Silvester Method:

1. Lay the casualty on his back on a firm surface with a rolled-up coat or something similar under his shoulders.

2. Kneel astride his head facing his feet. Grasp his wrists and cross them over the lower part of his chest.

3. Keeping your arms stiff, rock forward so that your weight presses down on the patient's chest. Maintain this pressure for a count of three.

4. Retaining your hold on the patient's wrists, rock backward, bringing his arms in a wide sweep upward and then outward as far as they will go.

5. Repeat the cycle rhythmically about 12 times a minute.

Painful breathing—May be due to something simple like "rheumatism" of the chest muscles (fibrositis) or something more serious like pleurisy. The majority of cases are not, however, due to pleurisy but to inflammation or injury.

You Should See Your Doctor If You Have Painful Breathing:

Within 12 hours If the pain is sharp or getting worse, or if it is accompanied by fever or cough.
Within 24 hours In all other cases.
What your doctor may do. He may make a particularly thorough examination of your chest and order a chest X-ray.
What you can do. Rest the muscles of your chest and shoulders as much as possible by avoiding heavy lifting. Heat from a hot water bottle or heat lamp and a gentle massage will be helpful. Aspirin or acetaminophen may be taken for the pain.
Shortness of breath (dyspnea)—Shortness of breath that is not the result of strenuous activity is a common and important symptom which should be taken seriously—not regarded as a consequence of "getting old." If walking up a hill or climbing a flight of stairs now makes you puff or stop to get your breath, you may have a disorder of the heart and respiratory system, or you may be too overweight. The breathlessness of heart disorders is often accompanied by swelling of the ankles (edema) and bouts of acute dyspnea when lying in bed at night (cardiac asthma or orthopnea). Dyspnea associated with a fever may be due to a respiratory infection, such as pneumonia; and wheezing with shortness of breath commonly occurs in attacks of asthma.

You Should See Your Doctor about Being Short of Breath:

Now If it comes on suddenly; if it is so severe that you are gasping; if it is accompanied by severe pain in the chest or coughing up fresh blood; if your face or fingers have become tinged with blue; or if it fails to respond to the drugs you usually take.

Within 12 hours If, for the first time or in spite of your usual medicine, it is severe enough to keep you in bed or is accompanied by fever, bloody phlegm, pain on breathing, or severe wheezing.

Within 24 hours If it is severe enough to prevent you from working or, in spite of your usual medicine, is much worse than usual; or if wheezing is persistent.

Within 7 days In all other cases.

What your doctor may do. The doctor will be particularly interested in the circumstances of the attack and will conduct a thorough examination of your heart and lungs. He may order a chest X-ray, heart tracing (electrocardiogram), or an assessment of your lung function (spirometry). Or he may refer you to a specialist.

What you can do. Often distressingly little. Try to sit rather than lie down and do something to distract yourself: read, listen to music, watch television. Don't pace restlessly around the room.

BRUISING

What you can do. Keep the part at rest until there is no danger of further bruising (about ten minutes). In the meantime, apply a cold compress. Soak a handkerchief or cloth in water as cold as you can get it; wring it out and place it on the bruised area. Bandage the compress in position and keep dripping cold water on it from time to time.

BURNS AND SCALDS

Burns are serious injuries because, quite apart from the amount of skin or other tissue that is destroyed, they are often accompanied by severe shock and extensive loss of body fluids from the exposed area. There also is a considerable risk of infection.

What You Can Do:

1. Put out the flames with cold water or smother them with a coat, rug, blanket, or towel; place these items toward the victim's feet to avoid driving the flames up into his face. Tear off smoldering clothes, gripping them by the nearest nonburning area. You may need to force the person to the ground to stop him from panicking and fanning the flames, but *do not* roll him around on the ground. Rolling will spread the flames and cause unnecessary additional burns.

2. Drench the burned area with cold water by holding it under the tap; by soaking it in a bowl, bucket, or bathtub; or by applying cold, wet cloths for at least ten minutes.

3. At the same time, remove any constrictive clothing, such as boots, bracelets, garters, or rings, before the burned area begins to swell.

4. Lay the patient down and keep him warm; shock can occur quickly and be severe.

5. Cover the burn with a light, moist, cold cloth or dressing. Do not touch the burned area with your fingers, burst any blisters, or apply lotions or creams.

6. Give sips of water or tea to replace the fluid lost through the burned area. (This is the one exception to the "nothing-by-mouth" rule in the care of victims of serious accidents.)

7. Get the patient to a doctor or hospital as quickly as possible for proper dressing of the burn and any other treatment that may be needed. Only very small burns can be managed safely without consulting your doctor. If the burn is small and you decide to treat it yourself, apply a generous amount of antiseptic cream to the area and cover with a dressing. If the burn is still painful after two days or in the process of becoming infected, get medical advice.

Chemical and hot-fat burns—These burns pose special problems. Both cause continuing damage if the clothes have been soaked in the corrosive substance. So the first priority is to remove your clothing. Chemical burns, in particular, must be thoroughly drenched in running water to remove all trace of the chemical. *Do not,* however, attempt to neutralize acid by applying alkali, or vice versa; this action will increase the damage to the skin. (See also the FIRE PLAN, pages 16–17.)

Sunburn—Calamine lotion, liberally applied, is as good as anything. If you are badly burned or think you may have sunstroke, you probably will need to see a doctor.

CHILLS

This term covers a multitude of conditions. Colds and influenza are the most common causes of chills, but chills also may be due to lengthy exposure to inclement weather (see EXPOSURE, pages 52–53). Shivering attacks usually are caused by a rapidly rising temperature as in feverish illnesses.

What you can do. Little can be done other than to keep the sufferer warm.

CHOKING

see BREATHING, Stopped, pages 31–34

COMA

see UNCONSCIOUSNESS, pages 97–98

CONSTIPATION

Constipation is the cause of a great deal of unnecessary, almost obsessive worry. Nobody ever met serious harm from it, and it is only rarely associated with serious disease. There is no natural law that states that the bowels should be moved at least once a day. Many people normally and happily do so once a week or even less often. And you will not be in danger of "poisoning your system" or any other problem if you miss a few days. The most common causes of constipation are a faulty diet and the habitual use of laxatives. Excessive laxative use makes the bowel expect the drugs and prevents it from acting without them. This condition is needless; yet millions of "laxative addicts" suffer from it every day.

Changes in the stool itself usually are not cause for concern. Alterations in the color, consistency, texture, or amount are probably the result of what you have been eating. Unless you have been taking iron, however, black stools (melena) are generally due to bleeding in the digestive tract. Watery stools may be due to colitis; thin, wormy stools may be due to a partial blockage in the bowel.

You Should See Your Doctor about Constipation:

Within 12 hours If it is accompanied by severe abdominal pain, persistent vomiting, or the eventual passage of a black stool.

Within 24 hours If it is accompanied by any abdominal pain or a bloated feeling (distension) in the abdomen or if you have had no bowel movements for four or more days.

Within 7 days If you have alternating constipation and diarrhea or a marked change in your normal bowel habits that has persisted for more than three weeks.

What your doctor may do. Your doctor will assess the extent of the problem from your account of it. He will examine your abdomen from the outside and the anal canal from the inside with a gloved finger. He will look into the anal canal with a small metal or plastic instrument (proctoscope) and a light. Neither of these examinations is as painful as you might expect. He also may order an X-ray of the bowel (barium enema).

What you can do. Make sure that you have enough fiber in your diet by eating plenty of whole-grain cereal foods. Change from white to whole wheat bread and from cooked to uncooked fruits and vegetables. Also get plenty of exercise. Don't resort to a laxative unless you have not moved your bowels for three days or are bloated and feel pain. If you do need to take a laxative, try a bulk-forming preparation, such as Epsom salts, twice a day. For more rapid action, you may try a bowel stimulant, such as senna (Senokot or Glysennid tablets). Take two tablets at bedtime; if they have no effect, take four tablets the following night. Senokot is also available in syrup form. Finally, you may insert a glycerol or bisacodyl suppository (Dulcolax). Above all, do not take laxatives for more than a few days without obtaining your doctor's advice. Don't take laxatives on a regular basis to "clean yourself out"; this is unnecessary and will do you far more harm than good.

CONVULSIONS

In children, convulsions are most likely due to high fever or to holding the breath too long. In adults, they usually are due to epilepsy or hysteria. In true epileptic convulsions, the patient lies still and is almost rigid for about a half-minute; then his body jerks uncontrollably for several seconds before he relaxes, resumes breathing, and slowly regains consciousness.

You Should See Your Doctor about Convulsions:

Within 24 hours If they have never occurred before or if they have never been investigated before.

What You Can Do:

1. *Do not* try to stop the convulsion by holding the patient still or by slapping his face.
2. Move the patient out of the way of anything that might injure him during his convulsion—a wall, heavy furniture, glass, or source of fire.
3. Try to remove false teeth, if present; clear any vomit out of the mouth; and wipe away froth.
4. Push a folded handkerchief, scarf, newspaper, or glove between the patient's teeth to prevent him from biting his tongue.

5. When the convulsion is over, lay the patient in the recovery position (see page 98).

6. In a child, if the convulsion is associated with a high fever, try to reduce the temperature by sponging the child with tepid (not cold) water or by giving him a tepid bath. If it is associated with a breath-holding incident, try to interrupt the action by making a sudden noise, such as banging on a table, slamming a door, or clapping your hands.

7. If the attack seems to be hysterical—that is, the patient is noisy, makes wild movements, and is aware of what everybody else is doing—be firm and reassuring but do not scold or ridicule. You may be wrong in your assessment of the situation. There is in any case something wrong with the patient.

COUGH

Although often a nuisance, coughing is one of the body's most effective protective mechanisms. It is designed to expel obstructive and unwanted material, such as phlegm (sputum) and foreign bodies, out of the lungs and the air passages. It often serves an important and useful purpose; so although a cough may be troublesome, you should think carefully before taking medicine that will diminish it. You may do yourself more harm than good by allowing heavily infected sputum to remain in your lungs where the phlegm will spread infection.

Coughs that produce sputum are called productive and should be encouraged; coughs that are dry serve no particularly useful purpose, are often painful and interfere with sleep, and can be safely suppressed. Some dry coughs arise from irritation in the back of the throat (in pharyngitis) or when mucus drips down from the back of the nose. It may be due to laryngitis or an infection in the windpipe (tracheitis). Sputum that is yellow or green is called purulent and usually is associated with such infections as bronchitis or pneumonia. Sputum that is clear and frothy is called mucoid and usually is associated with noninfective conditions.

You Should See Your Doctor about a Cough:

Now If a child's cough is croupy and accompanied by difficulty in breathing; or if a cough in a person of any age is associated with severe shortness of breath, pain in the chest, or bringing up fresh blood.

Within 12 hours If it is accompanied by any pain on breathing, bloody sputum, severe wheezing, shortness of breath, or a temperature over 102° F (39° C).

Within 24 hours If there is any wheezing, purulent sputum, or a temperature that has been above normal for more than four days.

Within 7 days In all other cases of persistent cough. A persistent cough is often the first indication of serious, but still curable, chest disease. Never go on hoping that it will go away or simply attribute it to smoking.

What your doctor may do. The doctor will thoroughly examine your chest, throat, and nose. He may order a chest X-ray, a special breathing test (spirometry), or laboratory tests on your sputum. He may prescribe cough medicine or antibiotics if there is evidence of a particular infection. He may feel that no treatment is likely to make any difference and therefore not prescribe anything.

What you can do. You can safely and effectively treat many coughs with the advice of your pharmacist. You should see your doctor, however, if any of the complications listed above arises or if your cough has not gone away within two weeks. For coughs due to mucus from the back of the nose (postnasal drip), use ephedrine or similar nose drops three or four times a day to dry up the secretion. Don't use these drops for more than five days without consulting your doctor. For coughs due to inflammation of the back of the throat and larynx, try inhaling menthol, eucalyptus, or other similar vapor several times a day (see page 10). Highly irritating, "throaty" coughs may be relieved by sucking cough lozenges. For dry coughs or for a cough that is seriously interfering with sleep, use a cough suppressant in doses of two teaspoons taken up to three times a day and once before bed. For coughs that cannot bring up sputum because it is too thick or sticky, use an expectorant. Dissolve the expectorant in a tumbler of hot water and sip it three or four times a day. You may want to take an expectorant during the day to help bring sputum up and a suppressant at night to quiet the cough so you can get to sleep.

CRAMPS

Cramps are painful muscle contractions that are rarely due to disease. They are likely to occur when muscles have gone into ,prolonged contraction (spasm).

What you can do. Cramps sometimes follow excessive sweating and then can be relieved by drinking a pint of water that contains a half-teaspoon of salt dissolved in it. In other cases, try to stretch the affected muscle. For cramps in the hand, straighten the fingers and bend them back. For cramps in the foot, push the toes upward. Bend the foot up and straighten the knee at the same time to ease cramps in the calf. Straighten the knee and pull the whole leg up or forward to ease cramps in the thigh. A cramp in the calf muscles that occurs with predictable regularity after walking a certain distance and then disappears almost immediately with rest is called *intermittent claudication*. It is a symptom of a circulation problem and should be reported to your doctor for further investigation since it often can be successfully treated.

CUTS

see WOUNDS, pages 104–5

DEAFNESS

The most common cause of deafness in young people is blockage of the ear canal by an accumulation of wax (cerumen). In elderly people, it is caused by degeneration of the hearing apparatus (presbycusis).

You Should See Your Doctor about Deafness:

Within 12 hours If it is accompanied by bleeding from the ear or pain.

Within 24 hours If it is accompanied by discharge from the ear or if it appeared suddenly.

Within 7 days In all other cases.

What your doctor may do. The doctor will look inside your ear with an instrument (otoscope) or a head mirror to find the cause of the deafness. If there is wax or other material in the ear, he may pick it out or remove it by syringing—squirting water into your ear to wash out the wax. These procedures are more alarming than painful. You may be asked to put drops or oil into your ear for a day or two beforehand to soften the wax so it will come out more easily (see page 11). If the deafness is not due to wax, your doctor may arrange to test your hearing (audiometry) and find out the degree and type of hearing loss you have. If your deafness is due to an infection, the doctor will prescribe an appropriate antibiotic. If he has doubt about the cause or management of your deafness, he may refer you to an ear specialist for further investigation.

What you can do. Do not try to remove earwax yourself—or let anybody else do it—even with something soft like cotton balls. You will press the wax further into the ear and probably increase your deafness. Even blunt objects can all too easily be pushed through the eardrum and thereby cause permanent deafness. Five drops of warm olive oil or Debrox placed in the ear three times a day for three days may soften the wax sufficiently for it to run out by itself. Do not attempt to syringe your own ears or anyone else's. If deafness persists for more than a few days or you feel that your hearing is less acute than before, consult your doctor soon. There are many ways in which you can be helped.

DEPRESSION

see EMOTIONAL AND MENTAL DISORDERS, page 51

DIARRHEA

Diarrhea means the frequent passage of loose or watery stools. It commonly is due to gastroenteritis or food poisoning. Serious diarrhea that accompanies general illness and abdominal pain may be due to dysentery or some other intestinal infection. Chronic diarrhea may be due to some form of inflammation or cancer of the colon, and even if it is not severe, it must not be allowed to continue for more than two weeks before seeing a doctor.

You Should See Your Doctor about Diarrhea:

Within 12 hours If your stools contain blood or you have severe abdominal pain.

Within 24 hours If it continues for more than two days (one day in a child) without improvement.

Within 7 days If you have repeated attacks, slimy or greasy stools, or concern about its seriousness.

What your doctor may do. The doctor will assess the extent of the problem from your account of it. He will examine your abdomen from the outside and perhaps the anal canal from the inside with a gloved finger or a small metal or plastic instrument (proctoscope) and a light. Neither procedure is as painful as you might expect. The doctor may send a stool specimen to a laboratory for examination. He may prescribe drugs to control the diarrhea but usually will not order antibiotics. Diarrhea commonly is caused by viruses, which are not affected by antibiotics. If diarrhea is persistent, the doctor may want to conduct further investigation in a hospital. He also may hospitalize patients with severe cases of diarrhea, particularly children.

What you can do. Most bouts of diarrhea can be safely and successfully treated without a doctor's help by obtaining medicine from the pharmacist. Kaolin in doses of four teaspoons dissolved in plenty of water may be taken every three or four hours until the diarrhea abates. Children may receive one teaspoon of kaolin every four hours if they are less than a year old, two teaspoons every four hours if they are between one and five years old, and four teaspoons every four hours if they are between five and twelve years old. Anyone suffering from diarrhea should drink plenty of fluids to replace those that are being lost. Take sips of cold water during acute stages of gastroenteritis; then try milk, bouillon, or other soup as the condition improves. If you are hungry, nibble a piece of dry toast or a plain biscuit; have cereal, rice, and pasta dishes as the diarrhea eases; and gradually work up to your usual diet. Don't persist with your own treatment for too long. If there has been no improvement in two days, see your doctor.

DISCHARGE

see the area of the body affected: ANAL, page 20; EAR, page 48; URETHRAL, page 98; VAGINAL, page 100

DIZZINESS

Giddiness (vertigo), faintness (syncope), and light-headedness are feelings which often are difficult to distinguish from one another. They may lead to unconsciousness (see page 97) and may be mistaken for convulsions (see page 40). They may be due to conditions that upset the usual operation of the brain—high blood pressure, anemia, hunger, prolonged standing, recent head injury, fever, physical or emotional shock. Or they may be due to disease of the organ of balance in the ear. Even if they occur several days apart, isolated attacks should be discussed with your doctor.

You Should See Your Doctor about Dizziness, Giddiness, Fainting, or Light-Headedness:

Now If full consciousness is not regained quickly; or if there are repeated attacks, especially after a recent injury to the head.

Within 12 hours If there are frequent attacks; if there have been similar attacks in the past; if there is any suspicion that the attack is some type of convulsion.

Within 7 days In all other cases.

What your doctor may do. The doctor will assess the nature of the problem from your description of it; your account of the way you felt during the attack is particularly important in pinning down the likely cause of the problem. The doctor may check your nervous system, ears, and eyes and will consider the possibility of anemia, increased blood pressure, diabetes, or epilepsy. He may order tests on the urine or blood or want you to see a nerve or ear specialist. He may want you to keep an eye on any subsequent attacks yourself and ask you to note their exact nature and the circumstances in which they occur. In the meantime, he may prescribe tablets to control the attacks.

What you can do. If you know that you are liable to get attacks of giddiness, move about deliberately and slowly. Particularly avoid sudden, sharp movements of your head. Spend a few moments sitting on the edge of the bed before rising in the morning and put your foot on a chair to tie your shoes rather than bend over. When possible, walk close to a wall or fence so you can lean on it if an attack occurs. Be particularly careful about driving or using machinery.

First Aid for Fainting

1. If there is room, lay the patient on the floor and hold his legs up so they are above the level of his head. If he is sitting or there is no room to stretch him out, push his head down between his knees and keep it there until the patient has fully recovered.

2. Loosen his collar and any other tight-fitting clothes. Splashing cold water on the face or using smelling salts may be helpful.

3. When he has recovered full consciousness, slowly raise him up and give him sips of cold water.

4. Do not leave him alone or let him try to walk for several minutes.

DROWNING

What You Can Do:

1. Get the casualty out of the water and preferably onto land. If this is not possible, get him into shallow water or a boat.

2. Quickly try to drain the water out of the lungs, but do not spend long doing it before starting artificial respiration. If the victim is a child, hold him up by his ankles and slap him hard between the shoulders for a few seconds. If the victim is an adult and you have room, lay him facedown in a slanted position with the head lower than the feet. Run two fingers around the inside of his mouth and throat to clear out any obstruction, such as seaweed or false teeth. After placing the victim facedown, thump him hard with the flat of your hand several times between the shoulder blades to provoke coughing or even breathing.

3. Immediately start artificial respiration, using the Holger-Nielsen or Silvester method (see pages 33–34). If he is in shallow water or a small boat and you cannot get him facedown, use mouth-to-mouth resuscitation (see pages 31–33). If you suspect that the heart has stopped beating, begin cardiac compression described on page 33.

EAR

Bleeding, see pages 26–27
Deafness, see page 44

Earache and **Ear Discharge** are most comonly due to infection in the inner part of the ear *(otitis media)*. An earache also may be caused by inflammation of other organs that share the same nerve supply, such as the molar teeth or the parotid gland (as in mumps). Pain and tenderness of the outer part of the ear or the ear canal most commonly is due either to a localized infection, such as a boil, or a type of eczema called *otitis externa*.

You Should See Your Doctor about an Earache or Ear Discharge:

Within 12 hours In all cases of discharge or pain from inside the ear, especially if accompanied by fever, pain behind the ear, or a headache.

Within 24 hours In all cases of pain or tenderness of the outer part of the ear.

What your doctor may do. The doctor will look inside your ear with an instrument (otoscope) or a head mirror to discover the cause of the pain or discharge. He may need to mop up the discharge with a cotton ball and may send a specimen to the laboratory for bacteriological tests. He also may look in your nose and throat because otitis media often results from infections that start there. He probably will prescribe an antibiotic to control the infection, tablets to relieve the pain, and perhaps a decongestant to decrease the amount of secretion from the inflamed tissues. He also may give you drops to put in your ear and drops to put in your nose to control congestion. He may refer you to an ear specialist for further investigation.

What you can do. Do not attempt to poke around in your ear or put drops into it unless instructed to do so by your doctor. Inhalants, such as menthol or eucalyptus, and decongestant tablets containing 60 mg ephedrine (Chlor-Trimeton) may be taken three times a day. But do not delay in seeing your doctor. In the meantime, hold a hot-water bottle against the ear and take two or three aspirin or acetaminophen tablets every three or four hours for the pain.

FOREIGN BODY IN THE EAR

What you can do. Turn the patient's head so the affected ear is pointed downward and gently shake it up and down. If you are lucky, the object will drop out. If the object does not drop out, take the patient to a doctor or hospital emergency department. *Do not* attempt to pry the object out, even with something blunt; you will likely cause serious damage. If the foreign body is an insect or something similar and the patient is sure that his eardrum was not perforated in the past, pour in a little tepid water or olive oil in the hope that the object will float out.

ELECTRICAL INJURIES

What You Can Do:

1. Attempt to remove the injured party from the source of the electricity but *take great care* or you may be injured, too. In the home, try to switch off the electricity, pull out the plug, or wrench out the cable without touching the patient. If this is not possible, try to knock or pull the patient clear of high-voltage equipment or power cables but make sure that you *do not touch the patient directly.* If possible, stand on dry, nonconductive material, such as a rubber mat, a coat, wood, or a pile of newspapers. Knock or pull the patient away from the electricity using a broomhandle, pole (never metal), piece of wood, cane (not umbrella), chair, rope, or rolled-up carpet.

2. Start resuscitation as described on pages 31–34.

3. Treat any burns as described on page 37.

When dealing with a victim who has been injured by extremely high voltages, keep clear, by at least twenty yards, until the current has definitely been switched off. The chance of doing anything useful for the victim is virtually nil; the chance of your being electrocuted if you attempt to get near him is very high.

EMOTIONAL AND MENTAL DISORDERS

Anxiety, depression, nervousness, stress, and more serious mental illness affect you or a close relative or friend. (See also pages 158–67.)

You Should See Your Doctor—or Persuade the Relative or Friend to See a Doctor:

Now If there is a strong compulsion or has been an attempt to commit suicide or to attack another person.

Within 12 hours If there are suicidal thoughts, severe depression, despair, or mental disturbance, such as delusions, hallucinations, or bizarre ideas.

Within 24 hours If depression, nervousness, tension, or any other mental disturbance makes going to work or school, or doing housework, impossible.

Within 7 days If there is insomnia that lasts more than four nights; undue nervousness, irritability, or aggressiveness; attacks of weeping; abnormalities of behavior, such as truancy, deception, or dishonesty; irrational or inappropriate ideas or reactions; serious worries about work or school, family or marriage, social or sexual relationships, money, housing, or some misdemeanor; excessive consumption of alcohol or drugs; a phobic or hysterical disorder.

What your doctor may do. The doctor will listen to your account of the problem and ask you questions to clarify or expand points that he has not understood or that seem to be important. He will discuss the situation as well as its implications and possible underlying features with you, and work out a practical plan of action for dealing with any factors in your job or homelife that may need to be changed. This plan may require cooperation with your family, friends, employer, priest or minister, social agencies, or housing authorities. The doctor may arrange for further consultations to delve more deeply into the problem and try to get at the root of the trouble and to assess your progress. If necessary, the doctor will prescribe drugs to calm or tranquilize you, counteract your depression, or help you sleep while your problems are being resolved. If the trouble is particularly complicated or deep-seated or you do not respond to treatment, he may refer you to a psychiatrist. If your state of mind is such that you are in danger of harming yourself or other people, he may arrange for your immediate admission to a hospital.

What you can do. Try to discuss work, marriage, money, social, sexual, or personality problems with somebody you trust as soon as they occur. Delay almost always leads to deterioration of the situation. Simply talking about problems—"getting them off your chest"—is surprisingly helpful; it eases the burden and diminishes the sense of pressure. It often makes a big difference to your insight into, and assessment of, the problem and can help you appreciate what is required to correct them. If talking about your problem is not enough, do not delay in seeing your doctor. The sooner emotional and mental problems are dealt with, the better; so don't wait until you are desperate. And don't delay because you feel that consulting your doctor about an emotional problem is a sign of weakness or failure or that he will regard you as a "mental" case or attribute all your subsequent illnesses to "nerves." He knows only too well, especially nowadays, that many factors affect people's illnesses. He probably has experienced depression himself and is well aware of what you are feeling.

EXPOSURE

Exposure to cold can affect the very young or the very old at home during the winter months or anyone who is out-of-doors for lengthy periods in excessive cold, dampness, and wind, such as sailors, hikers, and mountaineers. Exposure to cold leads to a considerable drop in body temperature. If the temperature drops below 95° F (35° C), the condition is called *hypothermia,* and it results in poor coordination, blurred vision, and slurred speech. Hypothermia often comes on gradually and may be unrecognized or mistaken for fatigue or general debility.

What You Can Do:

Out-of-doors—Protect the person against further heat loss. Get him into a sheltered spot and keep him there. Try to set up a cover or a windbreaker. Wrap the victim in blankets or put him in dry clothes and enclose him as completely as possible in a sleeping bag. Give him sips of a warm sweet drink. Get him back to base camp and into a warm bath as soon as possible, but *do not* use direct heat, such as a hot-water bottle or electric blanket. Frostbite is a particular hazard. Remove anything that fits tightly, such as a ring. Keep the frostbitten area warm and dry; cover the nose, chin, or ear with a gloved hand and put a frostbitten hand inside your clothes in an armpit. As soon as possible, *slowly* revive the frostbitten area with warm—never hot—water in a hot-water bottle or through direct exposure to a fire. *Do not* rub the area; rubbing will further damage the already fragile skin.

In-doors—Begin rususcitation if necessary (see page 31). Raise the body temperature *slowly* by wrapping the person in blankets, increasing the heat in the room, and giving the person sips of warm sweet drinks that contain a little brandy or rum.

EYE PROBLEMS

Eye problems may consist of pain, irritation, soreness, redness or inflammation, excessive watering, injury or bruising, "something in the eye," or some kind of disturbance or deterioration of vision.

You Should See Your Doctor about Your Eyes:

Now If there has been a serious injury or chemical burn or there has been sudden severe pain or loss of vision.

Within 24 hours If there is pain, soreness, redness, or irritation, or any discharge that is not watery; if the eyelids are stuck together on waking; if it hurts to look at bright lights; or if there has been a sudden deterioration in vision.

Within 7 days If there is persistent watering; if you see halos around lights; or if you have double, blurred, or otherwise disturbed vision.

You Should See an Optometrist or Ophthalmologist about Your Eyes:

If you believe your eyesight is not as good as it was, or if you are over age 40 and have not had your eyes checked in the past two years.

What your doctor may do. The doctor will assess the nature of the problem from your description of it. He will examine your eye and its movements and look into it with an instrument (ophthalmoscope). He will also test your sight and range of vision. If the problem is a straightforward one, he will prescribe eye drops or ointment and perhaps tablets. If not, he will refer you to an ophthalmologist or optometrist for further investigation or an assessment of the need for spectacles.

What you can do. Gently bathe the eye using a pint of warm boiled water with a level teaspoon of salt dissolved in it (see page 11). For comfort, cover the eye with a patch or pad made from layers of gauze. Avoid rubbing the eye. If there is no improvement the next day, see your doctor. *Do not* rely on over-the-counter preparations for eye problems.

FIRST AID TO THE EYE

Wounds to the Eye

What you can do. If anything is sticking into the eye, make
no attempt to get it out. Ask the patient to keep his eyes as
still as possible to avoid further damage. Covering the good
eye as well as the injured one will make this easier for him;
since the eyes move together, just as much damage may be
done by looking around with the good one. Cover the injured
eye lightly with a pad made from gauze.

Chemicals in the Eye

What you can do. Instant action is necessary. Place the
patient's head so the injured eye is to the side and down.
Immediately flood the eye with a steady flow of water or milk.
Pull the eyelids apart to make sure that any corrosive under
them is washed out. Keep rinsing the eye for ten minutes (by
the clock). Then cover the eye with a clean pad and send the
patient to a hospital.

Foreign Body in the Eye

What you can do. Keep the patient from rubbing the eye.
While the patient blinks rapidly, flood the eye with a steady
flow of water. If the object is in the center of the eye and has
not come out after washing, make no further attempt to
remove it. If it is not visible, sit down facing the patient and
slowly draw the lower eyelid outward and downward while he
looks upward. If you see the object, try to remove it using the
corner of a clean handkerchief. If it does not come away
easily, do not persist. If the object seems to be under the upper
lid, have the patient look down; then place a matchstick
across the upper lid. Grip the edge of the lid firmly, pull it
down and over the lower lid and then up over the matchstick.
If you see the particle, remove it. Wash out the eye after the

object has been removed. If the eye is still sore, cover it with a pad and send the patient to a hospital.

"Black-Eye"

What you can do. Apply a cold compress.

FAINTING

see DIZZINESS, pages 46–48

FATIGUE

Fatigue is defined as an overall lack of energy, weariness (as distinct from sleepiness), and a "run down" feeling. It is often associated with weakness, but a general feeling of weakness must be distinguished from weakness or loss of strength in a particular part of the body (see page 102). Fatigue is usual at the end of the day, after exertion, for several weeks after an illness or operation, during pregnancy and after childbirth, and in old age. Fatigue may be associated with a continuing infection that is not yet severe enough to make you obviously ill, such as tuberculosis, anemia, or a persistent loss of blood from heavy menstruation, inadequate nutrition, chronic liver or kidney disease, diabetes or thyroid disease, obesity, or cancer. In many cases, fatigue is due to an emotional disorder or boredom. Fatigue accompanied by loss of appetite and weight is a symptom of several serious conditions, and it should be investigated without delay. Fatigue may increase gradually without notice and may be attributed to being "run down" or "fed up" or a particular "time of life." Fatigue, consequently, may be ignored, tolerated, or dismissed as a sign of being weak-willed or as something too trivial to bother the doctor about. However, fatigue may be the first, and sometimes the only, indication of an underlying disorder that should be investigated and corrected. So if your fatigue does not abate within three or four weeks, discuss it with your doctor.

What your doctor may do. The doctor will assess the cause of fatigue from your account of the circumstances. Your description of what has been happening is particularly important. With it, the doctor can direct his examination to all the possible causes suggested by your account of the events. He may order urine and blood tests to check for the presence of diabetes, anemia, and other disorders. If the cause is not apparent, the doctor may refer you to a specialist for further investigation. He may suggest adjustments in your style of life or diet or prescribe drugs to provide temporary help. He probably will not give you stimulants or "pep pills." These drugs provide a short-term and completely artificial boost, cannot get to the heart of the problem, and may be addictive.

What you can do. Make sure that you are getting enough rest and relaxation and that your diet is adequate. If your diet is adequate, taking extra vitamins cannot possibly have any effect on your fatigue and can be dangerous. You would do yourself far more good by spending the money on a book.

FISH HOOK INJURIES

What You Can Do:

1. Clean the area with soap and water and, if possible, apply antiseptic. *Do not* try to drag the hook back through the skin.

2. Push the hook further forward until the point and the barb come out through the skin.

3. Using pliers or wire cutters, cut through the shaft of the hook. Then remove the eye and attached line.

4. Grip the point of the hook firmly and pull it out.

FLUSHING

As distinct from blushing, flushing is most commonly associated with a fever (see TEMPERATURE, page 94) or with the change of life (menopause) in women. Women with any menopausal symptoms should not tolerate them but ask a doctor for help.

FOREIGN BODIES

Some "foreign bodies" are driven into the body by force, such as bullets, shrapnel, or fragments of glass. Some are stuck into the flesh, such as splinters (see SPLINTERS, page 92), nails, and fish hooks (see FISH HOOK INJURIES, page 57), and cause wounds (see WOUNDS, page 104). Others get into natural body orifices, such as the ear or nose (see EAR, page 48; EYE, page 53; and NOSE, page 75).

What you can do. Do not attempt to remove objects that have penetrated into the flesh; this is a job for the experts. Foreign bodies in the throat often can be grasped and removed with the fingers. Those in the larynx or windpipe may be eliminated by coughing; you may give the patient a few sharp slaps on the back to provoke coughing. However, fish bones, pins, etc., usually require skilled removal. Complete obstruction of the windpipe is not common, but when blockage occurs, breathing is impossible and urgent action is necessary (see page 31). A foreign body in the esophagus that interferes with swallowing may be eliminated by pushing your fingers down the patient's throat to make him vomit. Often foreign bodies in the throat, windpipe, or esophagus scratch or inflame the lining of these body parts. For several days after the object was removed the scratch or inflammation may give the feeling that the object is still there. An amazingly large number of foreign objects that are accidentally or deliberately swallowed pass through the digestive tract without causing any trouble. If you think that you or your child has swallowed something unusual, there is seldom cause for alarm unless the object was sharp or there is sudden, severe abdominal pain or blood in vomit. In the absence of such symptoms, all you need do is watch the stools for a few days to make sure that the object reappears. If it does not, consult your doctor. He may order an X-ray to see where the object is. If it shows no sign of passing through by itself, the object may have to be removed by surgery. Children are liable, out of curiosity, to poke objects into any of their own or their friends' body orifices. Gentle attempts at removal are in order, but if the object does not come out easily, take the patient to the doctor or hospital emergency department.

FRACTURES

see INJURIES, pages 65–72

GIDDINESS

see DIZZINESS, pages 46–48

GLANDS

Swollen or tender glands may occur throughout the body, and the swelling may involve all the major groups of lymph glands—throat (tonsillar), neck (cervical), armpit (axillary), and groin (inguinal). Or the swelling may affect only one group of glands. The most common causes of general glandular enlargement (lymphadenopathy) are infectious diseases. Less common but more serious causes are syphilis, leukemia, and Hodgkin's disease. Enlargement or tenderness of a single gland or group of glands usually is due to an infection, such as a boil or cut in the vicinity of the gland that has become "septic" (lymphadenitis). Glands swollen from infection generally return to normal after the infection has subsided. Occasionally glandular enlargement may be due to the spread of previously unsuspected cancer.

You Should See Your Doctor about Swollen Glands:

Within 7 days If they have remained enlarged for more than a week or two.

What your doctor may do. The doctor will examine you to

search for possible causes, and he may order blood tests or refer you to a specialist for further investigation. If the cause of glandular enlargement is an infection, such as tonsillitis, a boil, or an infected wound, he probably will prescribe an antibiotic.

What you can do. Keep track of swollen glands by the calendar.

GRAZES

see WOUNDS, pages 104-5

HANGOVER

What You Can Do:

Drink plenty of water and, even if you don't feel like it, go for a brisk run. For throbbing or aching in the head, take two acetaminophen (Tylenol) tablets. For nausea or vomiting, take four teaspoons of a liquid antinauseant or a few antinauseant tablets, or drink a glass of milk.

HEADACHE

Headaches probably are the most common of all complaints. Occurring alone, a headache usually is caused by emotional stress or muscular tension in the head or neck. It also may occur in association with a wide variety of disorders, such as migraine, meningitis, high blood pressure, brain tumors, sinus disease, any feverish illness, and various toxic states, including a hangover.

You Should See Your Doctor about a Headache:

Now If severe drowsiness or unconsciousness develops.

Within 12 hours If there is slurred speech or difficulty in

using the arms or legs, severe vomiting, an
earache, or disturbances in vision; if bending
the neck is painful; or if there was a recent
injury to the head.

Within 24 hours If it is continuous, keeps you awake, or has
lasted for more than two days; if there is
giddiness, nausea or vomiting, an earache, or
a disturbance in vision.

Within 7 days If it has not gone away completely within
three days.

What your doctor may do. The doctor will assess the cause
of your headache from your description of it and the circumstances in which it occurred. He will examine you, paying
particular attention to the possible causes suggested by your
account of the events. He may check your eyes. In some cases,
he may order an X-ray of the skull or an examination of the
fluid in the spine (cerebrospinal fluid), which is obtained by a
lumbar puncture. (A lumbar puncture is unpleasant but not
as terrible as it sounds.) The doctor may refer you to a
specialist if he has any doubts about the cause of your
headache. He may prescribe a suitable drug to relieve the
pain, possibly in combination with a drug to relieve tension.

What you can do. Take two aspirin or acetaminophen
tablets every three or four hours, up to a maximum of twelve
a day. If possible, lie or sit down in a quiet, darkened room;
close your eyes; and rest your head on something. Massage the
back of the neck and scalp or apply a hot towel on the
forehead or the back of the neck.

HEAD INJURY

see INJURIES, pages 65–72

HEARTBURN

see INDIGESTION, pages 62–64

HICCUPS

Although annoying, hiccups rarely have any serious consequence. Most attacks last less than an hour, but you should
get help from your doctor if they continue for more than three
hours.

What you can do. There are many favorite remedies. Those
most likely to succeed include holding your breath as long as
possible, breathing in and out of a small bag, and making
powerful sucking movements while holding your breath.

HOARSENESS

Hoarseness is due to irritation of the vocal cords, and it is
commonly caused by inflammation of the voice box (laryngitis). It can, however, be due to a growth in the larynx.

You Should See Your Doctor about Hoarseness:

Within 7 days If it has lasted more than two weeks.

What your doctor may do. The doctor may refer you to a
throat specialist, who will be able to get a better look at your
larynx.

What you can do. Simple laryngitis from a cold, heavy
smoking, or overuse of the voice usually does not require
medical attention. Time and comparative silence, assisted by
inhalations of menthol and eucalyptus, are all that is necessary (see page 11).

HYPOTHERMIA

see EXPOSURE, pages 52–53

INDIGESTION

Indigestion may take many forms: dyspepsia, heartburn, acid
regurgitation, biliousness, flatulence, or a feeling of fullness in
the abdomen. And each indicates a stomach disorder. Most

attacks are due to excessive or ill-advised eating or drinking which causes inflammation of the stomach (gastritis). These attacks are .short-lived and respond to home treatment. Repeated or persistent attacks are probably due to stress or worry (nervous dyspepsia). Peptic ulcers and gall bladder disease are not common, and stomach cancers are unusual. They do occur, however; so you must not allow indigestion to continue more than two weeks, *even if it is relieved by over-the-counter medicine*, without consulting your doctor.

You Should See Your Doctor about Indigestion:

Now If you get sudden intense abdominal pain or vomit pure blood or heavily blood-stained or black vomit or material that looks like coffee grounds.

Within 12 hours If you have black or tar-like stools or vomit suspicious-looking material.

Within 24 hours If it is severe enough to keep you from working or sleeping or is accompanied by repeated vomiting; or if pain occurs in the back as well as the abdomen.

Within 7 days If it persists or you have repeated attacks for more than two weeks; if it fails to respond to medicine from the pharmacist; or if it is accompanied by nausea or vomiting.

What your doctor may do. The doctor will examine your abdomen. If the cause of the indigestion is straightforward, he will prescribe drugs, give dietary advice, and arrange to see you again for persisting or recurring trouble. If indigestion continues or returns, the doctor may change your treatment and arrange to see you again to assess its effect. At some stage, he may order an X-ray examination of the stomach (barium swallow) or gall bladder (cholecystogram), or he may refer you to a specialist for further investigation. If you have any bleeding in the stomach, he probably will arrange for you to be admitted to the hospital.

What you can do. Milk (not too cold), bicarbonate of soda dissolved in water, or some other household antacid are all suitable first aid measures. If you have a tendency to develop indigestion, you should be cautious about eating spicy foods and drinking coffee and alcohol. You should also avoid aspirin; take aspirin substitutes containing acetaminophen instead.

INFLAMMATION

Redness, tenderness, pain on use, and swelling can be due to infection, injury or "strain," or an allergic reaction. Inflammation, even though we regard it as unpleasant, is one of the body's most important defense and healing mechanisms. Thus, in most cases, it disappears by itself once its job is done. Inflammation often disappears in a few days. However, when muscles or ligaments are involved—in strains or sprains of the arms or legs and "rheumatism" of the chest (fibrositis)—it may last as long as several weeks. If an inflammation continues to spread or gets more intense two days after it began or it shows little or no signs of improvement in four days, consult your doctor.

What you can do. Treatment of inflammation depends on the underlying cause, but this is one condition about which you can do a great deal for yourself. Time is the major healer here, but there are many ways in which you can help. Of these, rest is the most important. Don't use the affected part of the body more than is absolutely necessary; protect and support the area with cotton padding and a firm (but not tight) bandage; if necessary, immobilize the inflamed part of the body in a sling or some kind of splint. Heat is also useful both to increase the blood supply to the affected part and to relieve the pain. Heat usually is applied in a compress or poultice, but make sure the compress or poultice is not hot enough to burn your skin. Use of a liniment or balm should be left until you are sure of the cause of the inflammation. Liniments and balms are helpful in the treatment of strains and inflammation of muscles, but they aggravate and are potentially dangerous in the treatment of inflammation due to infection. Simple pain-killing drugs, such as aspirin or acetaminophen may be taken two or three at a time in intervals of three or four hours. Inflammation also can occur internally, and it is covered later in the book in relation to the particular organ or part of the body that is affected.

INJURIES

Injuries to special organs, such as the EYE are dealt with under the appropriate heading. Specific injuries, such as BLEEDING (page 25), BRUISING (page 36), BURNS (page 36), WOUNDS (page 104), and ELECTRICAL INJURIES (page 50), are dealt with separately. The effects of injury to the body vary from simple, minor damage, such as a strain or sprain, to complex and serious damage involving fractures or crushed organs. In the first moments after an accident, the exact nature of the injuries or how serious or extensive they are often are not easy to determine. In case there is more damage than seems likely at first—an underlying fracture, for instance, may appear to be only a sprain—it is always wise to err on the side of caution. Never forget, either, that whatever the particular injuries may be, an injured person is likely to develop shock, and shock will more likely have fatal consequences than even highly extensive injuries.

What You Can Do:

Treatment of minor or major injuries follows the same general principles. Use your common sense to modify these principles according to the place and nature of the accident, the part of the body affected, and the probable severity of the damage.

1. Do not move the casualty unless he is in danger; treat him on the spot (see the section on first aid, pages 13–14).

2. When moving the injured part, support it firmly from

underneath at the site of the injury—not on either side of it—
to avoid any further displacement of possibly broken bones.

3. Try to control bleeding (see BLEEDING, page 25).

4. Cover wounds with as clean a cloth as possible (see
WOUNDS, page 104). *Do not* interfere with or attempt to
remove foreign bodies or protruding bones.

5. Immobilize and rest the injured part as well as you can.
The patient's own body is often the best splint; so bandage a
broken leg to the sound leg or secure a broken arm against the
chest with a sling. Other emergency splints can be made from
pieces of wood or rolled up cardboard or newspapers. Make
sure that emergency splints are wide enough to give adequate
support and long enough to immobilize the joints immediately above and below the injury. Put on plenty of
padding—towels, newspapers, fabric—between the skin and
the splint. Bandage the splint firmly but not tightly enough to
interfere with the circulation and take care not to put bandages or tie knots over the site of the injury. Emergency
bandages can be made from scarves, ties, stockings, etc. (For
further details on bandaging, see pages 109–10.)

6. Take steps to prevent shock (see SHOCK, page 89).

7. Do not do more than is absolutely necessary before
getting medical help.

First Aid for Strains

1. Check for underlying fractures.

2. If there are none, massage the area for 15 minutes, 4
times a day. (For further details on massages, see page 111.)

3. At other times, apply heat and give additional support to
the part with a firmly applied elastic bandage. (For further
details on the use of heat, see page 110).

First Aid for Sprains

1. Check for underlying fractures.

2. If the sprain has just occurred, soak the area in a basin of cold water or apply a cold compress. Cold applications reduce the swelling and bruising that occur immediately after a sprain; they have no effect on already developed sprains.

3. Bandage the joint firmly in the most comfortable position and use plenty of padding. If the ankle is injured, do not take off the shoe; the shoe provides considerable support and may be difficult to get on again. If the wrist, elbow, or shoulder are injured, a sling may be necessary.

First Aid for Dislocations

1. Immobilize the area in the most comfortable position.

2. Do not attempt to correct the dislocation; you may do far more harm than good.

First Aid for Fractures

1. If you think there is a possible fracture, treat it as if it is an actual fracture.

2. Follow the procedure for treating injuries (pages 65–66).

(For details on the management of fractures at particular sites, see the following pages.)

Crushing injuries—When a limb has been crushed for an hour or more by a heavy weight, such as a vehicle, machinery, or rubble from a collapsed building, there may be no outward sign of injury but considerable internal damage to muscles, bones, blood vessels, and nerves. Once the victim is released, however, the damaged area may swell rapidly, and the patient may develop severe shock.

First Aid for Crushing Injuries

1. Free the crushed limb as quickly as possible, but with great care.

2. Support the limb so the fingers or toes are above the rest of the body. Apply a broad elastic bandage in an overlapping spiral; try to cover the entire limb from the wrist or ankle to the shoulder or hip.

3. If the victim is conscious and has no internal injuries, give him a pint of fluid to drink at once. Later, give him regular sips of liquid to replace the fluid that has been lost from the blood vessels into the swollen tissue and to avoid a critical fall in blood pressure.

Head injuries—A concussion may occur and damage the brain even if the skull has not been fractured. The casualty may want to get up and walk away without any further fuss as soon as he regains consciousness. This should be strongly discouraged; even a temporary loss of consciousness calls for a full medical examination of the skull to learn the extent of any internal damage. In addition, all victims of head injuries should be carefully watched—by somebody in the family or a friend—for at least two days. Damage inside the skull may develop gradually; a torn blood vessel may leak very slowly or a fragment of bone may slowly start to press on the brain. The victim may not lose consciousness or regain it quickly and be alert for many hours before the damage inside the skull begins to affect him. However, if something is not done about that damage quickly, the victim may die or suffer permanent brain damage. No matter how minor, drowsiness or lack of concentration, nausea and vomiting, disturbances in vision, and irregular breathing, which occur within hours or days of a head injury indicate internal damage. A fracture at the base of the skull may be revealed through bleeding from the ear or nose or bruising around the eye.

First Aid for Head Injury

1. If the victim is or becomes unconscious, treat him as described on pages 97–98.

2. If not, keep the patient lying down and as calm as

possible until a doctor or ambulance arrives. Explain to him why this is necessary.

3. Run a finger around the inside of his mouth to make sure that the airway is clear. Check for bleeding from the ear or nose and for injuries in other parts of the body, especially the spine.

4. Check regularly, and if possible keep a written record of, the victim's breathing and pulse rates; the state of his pupils (large or small, equal or unequal); and other features, such as changes in the level of consciousness, vomiting, jerking of limbs, etc.

First Aid for Fractured Jaw

1. If he is not otherwise injured, the casualty may feel most comfortable holding the jaw up with his hands.

2. If he is not comfortable this way, you may splint the lower jaw to the upper jaw by placing a bandage under the chin, running one end of it across the top of the head and down to just above the ear on the opposite side, then crossing over the other end of the bandage, forming a band around the crown of the head, and tying off the bandage above the other ear.

Spinal injuries—A panicky or overenthusiastic bystander can do serious and irreparable harm to victims of spinal injuries. So your major task is to prevent anybody from trying to move or interfere with the victim before skilled help arrives. Persuade the victim to keep still; even slight movements of fractured spinal bones can enormously increase the damage to the spinal cord. A person with a serious back injury should be moved only to get him out of the way of even greater danger to his life—from cars on a busy highway or from debris from a collapsing building. If a victim must be moved, try to give total support to the entire body, preferably with the help of at least three other people. With the victim's head supported and legs tied together, roll him onto a padded gate or door, blanket or overcoat. This "stretcher" should be kept as taut or rigid as possible while all four people move simultaneously. You may gently insert a finger into the victim's mouth to remove any obstruction if you see that his airway may be blocked.

Chest injuries—Damage may have been done to the spine, heart, lungs, or ribs. Injury or fracture of the ribs alone is more painful and frightening than serious, and it seldom requires any special action.

First Aid for Chest Injury

1. In case the spine has been damaged, do not move the victim (see above).

2. If not, support the victim in a semi-upright position, but leaning toward the injured side, on pillows or coats with something firm, such as a wall or the wheel of a car, at his back.

3. Check that the airway is clear by running a finger around the inside of the mouth. Loosen any restrictive clothing.

4. Dress any wounds but do not try to remove any objects that have penetrated the chest; air sucked into the chest through such a wound can dangerously interfere with breathing. Try to seal chest wounds by squeezing the edges together with your fingers or by putting the flat of your hand firmly across the hole until you can make an airtight plug from a dressing and strap it firmly in position.

5. Remember to watch for, and try to prevent, shock (see SHOCK, page 89).

Fractured Collar Bone (Clavicle)

1. Support the elbow on the injured side.
2. Place a soft, bulky pad under the armpit.
3. Gently bend the elbow and move the arm up until the patient can hold onto his opposite shoulder.
4. Increase support to the injured side with an arm sling.

Abdominal injuries—Crushing injuries, strong blows, and

penetrating wounds may damage one of the many abdominal organs.

First Aid for Abdominal Injury

1. In case the spine has been damaged, do not move the victim (see *Spinal injuries,* page 69).

2. If not, lay the victim down with his head turned to one side. Put a pillow or rolled-up coat under his neck and another under his knees. Keep him as quiet as possible. *Do not* give him anything to eat or drink.

3. Cover any wounds. *Do not* attempt to remove any foreign objects or to replace any loops of intestines or other organs that may be sticking out. Be sure the dressing is large enough to amply cover the hole on all sides so there will be no further protrusion of abdominal contents. Firmly secure the dressing, but do not press down too hard.

4. If the lower abdomen or pelvis has been damaged, there is a chance that the bladder has been damaged. Ask the victim to try to avoid passing urine.

5. If the victim has difficulty or feels pain when he tries to move his thighs or trunk, the pelvic bones may have been damaged. In this case, bandage the legs firmly together after placing a padding of coats or cushions between them.

6. Remember to watch for and try to prevent shock (see SHOCK, page 89).

First Aid for Arm Fractures

1. Try to bend the victim's elbow.

2. If bending is painful, keep the arm straight and splint the whole arm. Bandage the arm to a board or plank or to the side of the body.

3. If bending is not painful, put a pad in the armpit, bring the forearm across the chest, and bandage the forearm in place with an arm sling.

4. In cases of crushing injury or suspected fracture of the

bones of the hand, the injured hand should first be supported—if necessary, by the patient himself using the palm of his other hand—and as soon as possible placed, well padded, in an arm sling.

First Aid for Leg and Foot Fractures

1. If the injured leg is lying at an unusual angle, do not attempt to move it; the fracture is probably complicated, and movement could increase the damage.

2. Otherwise slowly and gently try to bring the sound leg and the injured one in line with one another.

3. After placing padding, such as coats or pillows between the legs, bind the ankles and feet together by making a figure-eight bandage. Then bind the knees together.

4. Serious injury to the knee is best dealt with by immobilizing the entire leg. Place a board or plank behind the leg and bind the board to the leg.

5. In cases of a crushing injury or a possible fracture of the bones of the foot, remove the shoe and sock to assess the extent of the damage and dress any wounds and to avoid constricting the foot as it swells. A badly injured foot tends to swell rapidly, and unless removed soon, the shoe may have to be cut off. Place a padded splint on the sole of the foot and secure the splint with a figure-eight bandage if necessary later.

INSOMNIA

see SLEEPLESSNESS, pages 90–91

ITCHING OR IRRITATION (PRURITUS)

Itching may occur all over the body, particularly if you have taken food or a drug to which you are allergic, if you have diabetes, liver or kidney disease, or if you are anxious or stressed. Itching may occur only in certain areas following a sting or bite or in association with urticaria, eczema, or some other form of dermatitis, a fungal infection of the skin such as athlete's foot, or chilblain. Itching is often short-lived and goes away by itself. If it persists for more than a week or two, consult your doctor. After a week or two, itching will become very annoying, and it can be an indication of a serious underlying disease.

What you can do. Apply calamine lotion or cream and try to identify the cause of the irritation. Avoid scratching as much as you can.

LUMPS

Lumps can occur on any part of the body, and they may be due to inflammation, an accumulation of fluid, or a growth. Most people quite understandably find the development of a lump very worrying because it may turn out to be cancer.

You Should See Your Doctor about a Lump:

Within 7 days In all cases.

MENSTRUAL PROBLEMS

Absent or ceased periods (amenorrhea) are commonly related to pregnancy, breast feeding, change of life (menopause), emotional upsets, or hormonal disorders. Frequent (polymenorrhea), heavy (menorrhagia), prolonged or irregular periods are commonly related to inflammation in the womb or fallopian tubes, abnormal pregnancy, fibroids, ovarian cysts, intrauterine contraceptive devices, harmless and cancerous tumors, and emotional upsets. Painful periods (dysmenorrhea) commonly occur without any particular cause. They are, however, more likely to develop in relation to anxiety or worry of a sexual origin, inflammation of one or more of the pelvic organs, or an abnormally placed womb. Many of these conditions are not serious, but a few are; so you should not let menstrual problems continue for more than two cycles without seeing your doctor. You should see a doctor even sooner if you are over age 40 and have menstrual irregularity and particularly if bleeding returns—even for only a few hours—after you thought that you had gone through menopause. In most cases, such bleeding is not due to anything serious. It could, however, warn of cancer while the disease is still curable. If you ignore this warning, you may lose your chance for a cure.

You Should See Your Doctor about Menstrual Problems:

Within 7 days If bleeding returns—for only a few hours—after completion of menopause.

What your doctor may do. The doctor will assess the cause of your menstrual problems from your account of them and may ask questions about your private life. He will make a surface examination of your abdomen and an external and internal examination of your vagina and pelvic organs. He will insert a plastic or metal instrument (vaginal speculum) into your vagina so he can see clearly. (The procedure is unpleasant but not usually painful.) He may take material from the vagina or the neck of the womb for analysis in the laboratory. If indicated, he may arrange for a pregnancy test. He may recommend an operation to examine the womb called a D & C (dilation and curettage). The doctor may, however, need none of these examinations to find the cause of the problem.

What you can do. Keep an accurate record of all vaginal bleeding, lower abdominal pain, and sexual activities. For menstrual pain, take two or three aspirin or acetaminophen tablets every four hours up to a maximum of twelve a day. If you do not find them to be adequate, consult your doctor.

MENTAL

see EMOTIONAL AND MENTAL DISORDERS, page 51

NAUSEA
see VOMITING, pages 101–2

NERVOUSNESS
see EMOTIONAL AND MENTAL DISORDERS, page 51

NEURALGIA

In a sense, all pain is felt in the nerves, but some pain particularly involves nerves. Pain involving nerves occurs when a nerve is inflamed (neuritis), such as in shingles (herpes zoster), or when a nerve has been subjected to pressure or irritation, as in sciatica. The pain of neuralgia can be persistent and disturbing, and you may need to see your doctor for something stronger than aspirin or acetaminophen as well as for investigation of the problem.

NOSE
see BLEEDING, page 27

Foreign body—Do not try to poke the object out. Determine in which side of the nose the object has become lodged. Then pinch the opposite side of the nose closed, take a deep breath, and while keeping your mouth closed, snort out as hard as you can through the other nostril. If the object has not come out after the third attempt, sniff some warm water up the obstructed nostril and try again. If you still have no success, go to your doctor or the hospital emergency department.

Running (rhinorrhea)—A running nose may be due to infection, such as the common cold or sinusitis; allergic conditions, such as hay fever or other types of allergic rhinitis; the presence of a foreign body; or anxiety or stress. In many cases, it will be accompanied by sneezing. A running nose that has persisted for more than a week or two should be investigated and treated by your doctor.

What you can do. You may try to relieve a running nose by inhaling menthol or eucalyptus (see page 11). If a running or blocked nose interferes with your work, you may use a nasal spray or drops. Drops containing ephedrine are as good as any (see page 11).

PAIN

As an enemy of medicine, pain is third only to death and disability. It is to be avoided or counteracted whenever possible and often regardless of the cost. Pain is the result of the body's alarm system. It is the consequence of a disruptive jangling of the nerves that warns us something is wrong.

Assessment of the significance of pain is not easy. The emotional climate surrounding the situation and a person's usual response to discomfort and adversity determine his "pain threshold." An individual's pain threshold substantially affects the amount of pain he feels regardless of the severity of the physical disorder that gives rise to it. Nevertheless, we do attempt to assess the significance of the pain we feel, and we make mistakes. First, we understandably assume that the site of the pain indicates which organ or part of the body is diseased or injured. However, without some knowledge of anatomy, we easily can be mistaken about the position of organs in the body and about the location of pain arising from a particular organ. For instance, many people who are concerned about a possible heart problem report pain in a part of the chest which is not associated with the heart. Also, pain often arises in one place but is felt somewhere else along the same set of nerves. Disease in the gall bladder, for instance, causes pain in the right shoulder.

Assessment of the type and severity of pain also is important. Pain may be shooting or stabbing. It may be continuous or come and go. The symptoms that accompany pain, such as bleeding, swelling, or a disturbance in function, obviously help interpret the seriousness of its cause. Another clue is the timing of the pain. Severe pain of sudden onset probably signals a serious event that requires prompt medical attention. As for the severity of pain, although classifying a subjective and variable feeling is admittedly difficult, we must have some scale by which to relate the degree of pain to the seriousness of the underlying disorder and the need for quick action. For this purpose, pain is graded into four categories. The categories do not necessarily refer solely to the severity of the pain but to all the factors that indicate the importance of the underlying disease.

You Should See Your Doctor about New Pain:

Now For **** (4-star) pain; that is, pain that occurs suddenly and is so severe that you collapse, have to stop whatever you are doing, or need to call out for help; or severe pain that is accompanied by bleeding from any source or the loss of use or feeling in any part of the body. Unless a doctor is immediately available, get somebody to telephone for an ambulance to take you to a hospital.

Within 12 hours For *** (3-star) pain; that is, pain that is bad enough to make you stop work and go home.

Within 24 hours For ** (2-star) pain; that is, pain that is bad enough to keep you from sleeping or awakens you; pain that returns repeatedly; or pain that is associated with other symptoms, such as vomiting, jaundice, a bowel disorder, fever, etc.

Within 7 days For * (1-star) pain; that is, in all other cases.

What your doctor may do. The doctor will assess the cause of the pain from your description of it and the circumstances in which it developed. He will examine you, concentrating on the possible causes suggested by your account of the events. He may refer you to a specialist for further investigation. As soon as possible, he will give you something for the pain, by injection if it is very severe, or in tablets. The doctor sometimes cannot provide drugs for immediate relief, even to somebody in severe pain, because he must make sure he knows exactly what is wrong with you, and powerful painkilling drugs substantially alter the evidence on which he has to work. So in the long-term interests of the patient's eventual recovery, the doctor can give no painkilling drugs until the situation has been fully assessed.

What you can do. Don't put up with pain, especially new pain, just to show how brave or strong-willed you are; you probably will end up taking it out on people close to you by being irritable or depressed. And remember, medicine puts no premium on unnecessary endurance tests. Pain is designed to be an alarm that you ignore at your peril. Since you'll have to see your doctor about it sooner or later, you may as well see him sooner—within the next week at the most—and save yourself the worry of uncertainty and the risk of missing the chance for a cure. By all means, take over-the-counter painkillers (two aspirin or acetaminophen tablets every four hours up to a maximum of twelve a day). But if they don't relieve the pain, prevent it from returning, or get rid of the pain in three days, then you have something your doctor should know about. Also try to keep yourself busy. Pain seems to be much worse at night because our minds are not occupied. The ability to concentrate on something—music, art, reading, television—can help deal with pain.

Pain also must be considered in relation to the part of the body in which it is felt.

Generalized pain—Which is felt all over the body, may be associated with an infection such as a cold or influenza; unaccustomed use of muscles; rheumatic fever; or widespread arthritis. Such pain will get better by itself in a few days or respond to the home treatment suggested above.

You Should See Your Doctor about Generalized Pain:

Within 24 hours If a fever and the pain make use of any joint impossible or very difficult; if there is a rash or fever of over 104° F (40° C); or if a fever has persisted for more than four days.

Abdominal pain—Can be due to a great many disorders. Continuous pain over the entire abdomen which occurs suddenly and is intense enough to make you feel faint, interfere with your breathing, and make you fearful of imminent death is likely due to peritonitis. Peritonitis that is caused by the rupture of an infected appendix or peptic ulcer brings on * * * * pain; peritonitis that is caused by the spread of inflammatory material into the abdominal cavity from the womb or gall bladder usually elicits * * * pain. Pain of * * * intensity that comes and goes in waves—with build-up, peak, and fade-away phases—probably is due to a spasm in a small tube that is trying to squeeze something out, such as the kidney or gall bladder trying to get rid of stones, or to inflammation of a tubular organ, such as the appendix or colon. Aching * * pain is usually due to inflammation of one of the abdominal organs. Its accompanying symptoms indicate which organ may be involved.

You Should See Your Doctor about Abdominal Pain:

Now If it is * * * * pain or if it is intense; if it makes you writhe, feel faint, or become very ill; if it is accompanied by vomiting pure blood or heavily blood-stained, black, or coffee ground-like material; or if it occurs within two days of an abdominal injury.

Within 12 hours If it is * * * pain; if it comes in waves with build-up, peak, and fade-away phases; if it is accompanied by black or tar-like stools or an inability to urinate; or if it occurs in someone who is, or may be, pregnant.

Within 24 hours If it is ** pain; if it is accompanied by nausea, vomiting, diarrhea, fever, rash, jaundice, painful or frequent urination or abnormal vaginal bleeding or discharge.

Within 7 days If it is * pain; or if it persists, returns, or fails to respond to home treatment.

What your doctor may do. The doctor will thoroughly examine your abdomen to find out the cause of the trouble. The examination may cause you additional pain as he presses on the areas that hurt, but the pain cannot be avoided. The doctor will, of course, be as gentle as possible. If necessary, he will refer you to a specialist for further investigation. As soon as possible, the doctor will prescribe drugs to relieve the pain.

What you can do. For abdominal pain of any severity, you can do very little except get medical attention as quickly as your symptoms indicate. Avoid eating or drinking anything in case you may need an operation. Hot-water bottles or an electric blanket or heating pad laid across the abdomen will give you some relief.

Anal pain—see pages 20–21

Back pain—Back pain has many causes, some involving the spine itself. The common causes are injury to the spine from consistently poor posture or a simple strain, a displaced or "slipped" intervertebral disc, a crush fracture, or chipping of the bones of the spine and degenerative changes, such as osteoarthrosis or spinal arthritis. A rare cause is the spread of cancer or an infection, such as tuberculosis or osteomyelitis. Conditions which are not directly related to the spine but which may give rise to backache include severe peptic ulcers, disorders of the kidneys, bladder, or womb, and menstrual problems.

You Should See Your Doctor about Back Pain:

Now If it is **** pain; or if it is accompanied by the loss of use or feeling in any part of the body or by the inability to urinate.

Within 12 hours If it is *** pain; if it is accompanied by bleeding or pain on urination or difficulty or pain on breathing; or if there has been an injury to the back.

Within 24 hours If it is ** pain; or if it is accompanied by fever, irregular vaginal bleeding or vaginal discharge, abnormal menstrual cycles, or pain in the thigh or leg.

Within 7 days In all other cases of new or unexplained back pain.

What your doctor may do. The doctor will examine your back, chest, abdomen, and limbs and the nerves relating to them. He may order special tests on your urine and X-rays of the painful part of your back. If the cause is a disorder of the spine, such as lumbago, a strain, sciatica, or arthritis, he will prescribe a suitable rest and exercise regimen and the use of heat and massage at home. If this plan does not relieve the pain, he will arrange for you to have physical therapy. He also will prescribe appropriate painkilling and muscle-relaxing drugs.

What you can do. Nonserious conditions that cause low back pain often respond well to home treatment involving rest, exercise, heat, and massage (see page 110). If you have sudden back pain, try to lie down as flat as you can or to hang by your hands from the top of a door. After the crisis has passed, rest, flat on your back, on a firm surface, such as a plank or a door or even on the floor until you are free of pain. You may continue to feel pain for as little as two or three days or as much as two or three weeks. Once you are free of pain, you can begin exercises prescribed by your doctor and designed to rehabilitate and strengthen the back muscles and ligaments. Do a little more each day but always stop when you begin to feel pain; to persist beyond this point may cause a flare-up of your problem.

Painful breathing—see page 35

Chest pain—Chest pain must always be taken seriously. You should, however, resist the temptation to conclude that you have a heart condition. A heart condition is not the most common cause of chest pain. Believing that your chest pain means you are having a heart attack can, in itself, do considerable harm. Persistent, **** pain in the center of the chest beneath the breastbone that feels as though you are held in a vise, spreads down into the left arm, and is accompanied by faintness or collapse is associated with a heart attack or coronary thrombosis. After a heart attack, many people have heart pain *(angina)*. Angina usually is not so severe. It occurs after physical exertion or excitement and is relieved by rest or by a tablet of nitroglycerine placed under the tongue. Tenderness over part of the chest and pain that occurs when moving the shoulders or arms are more common than heart pain. Both symptoms are muscular in origin and are due to a strain or an inflammation of fibrous tissue *(fibrositis)*. Pain while breathing or coughing may be an indication of pleurisy, but it is more likely due to an injury to the chest that has strained the chest muscles or damaged the ribs. Persistent aching that is accompanied by a rash on one side of the chest only indicates shingles *(herpès zoster)*. Digestive disorders, heartburn and other types of dyspepsia, and disorders of the shoulders or upper spine also may give rise to pain in the chest.

You Should See Your Doctor about Chest Pain:

Now If it is **** pain; or if it is accompanied by faintness, sweating, shortness of breath, or vomiting blood.

Within 12 hours If it is *** pain; if it makes breathing very uncomfortable; or if it is accompanied by an irregular pulse.

Within 24 hours If it is ** pain, if it occurs during exertion or excitement; if it is accompanied by persistent vomiting, a rash on the chest, or a fever; or if it follows an injury to the chest or lower back.

Within 7 days If it persists for, or returns within, two days.

What your doctor may do. The doctor will assess the cause of the pain. He will rely on your description of what you felt and when you felt it. Your description is extremely important because an examination may not turn up anything definite. The doctor will check your pulse and blood pressure and look for disorders in the chest. In some cases, he may arrange for an electrocardiogram (ECG), an X-ray of the chest, and an X-ray of the esophagus (barium swallow). He will give an injection or tablets to relieve the pain as soon as possible. He may refer you to a specialist for further investigation and treatment.

What you can do. Don't get yourself into a "heart attack" frame of mind. Pains in the chest that are related to movement or accompanied by tenderness at the site of the pain can be treated at home with rest, exercise, heat, and massage (see page 110). If you are uncertain or worried about the cause of the pain or the pain does not respond to home treatment within five days, go to your doctor. Two aspirin or acetaminophen tablets every four hours up to a maximum of twelve a day usually are effective in controlling pain.

Ear pain—see EAR, pages 48–50

Eye pain—see EYE, pages 53–56

Face pain—Infected teeth, sinus inflammation (sinusitis), mumps, blows, facial neuralgia (trigeminal neuralgia or tic douloureux), and inflammation of the blood vessels in the temple (temporal arteritis) are the common causes of facial pain. If the pain does not improve with treatment at home (aspirin or acetaminophen or inhalants for sinusitis [see page 9]) within two or three days, consult your doctor.

Head pain—see HEADACHE, pages 60–61

Pain on intercourse (dyspareunia)—May be due to physical causes, such as inflammation of the genital organs, or to emotional difficulties. In either case, if pain occurs on more than three occasions, go to your doctor as soon as possible. Delay can give rise to other problems.

Joint pain and muscle pain—Although they can occur separately, joint and muscle pain often go together to make up what is generally known as rheumatism. Overuse, strain, poor posture, and short-lived viral infections are the most common causes. More serious infections, such as rheumatic fever, bone diseases, rheumatoid arthritis, osteoarthritis, or gout, also may be the cause of the pain. No form of rheumatism should be allowed to continue indefinitely without investigation in the mistaken belief that it will get better eventually or that little can be done for it anyway. Make up your mind that if your rheumatism has not improved *within two weeks* (by the calendar), you will see your doctor about it.

What you can do. A combination of rest and exercise, heat and massage (see page 109), and aspirin or acetaminophen tablets taken every three or four hours up to a maximum of twelve a day will help.

Neck pain—Most pain in the muscles and joints of the neck is due to strain or tension, and sometimes it is accompanied by stiffness. Pain and stiffness usually respond to treatment at home (see page 109). The great concern with neck pain is that it might be due to meningitis. Meningitis causes severe headache, fever, and a sensitivity to bright light in addition to neck pain and stiffness that is so severe the patient cannot touch his chest with his chin. Nevertheless, if you are in doubt, see your doctor without delay.

Painful periods—see MENSTRUAL PROBLEMS, pages 73–74

Shoulder pain—This very common condition can be due to injury or strain, excessive or unbalanced use (too heavy a load carried on one side), poor posture, or disorders of the neck joints or muscles.

What your doctor may do. The doctor may order an X-ray of the shoulder to rule out a serious problem and start you on a course of physical therapy. In some cases, the doctor may give an injection directly into the joint.

What you can do. A combination of rest and exercise, heat and massage (see page 109) is often effective.

Pain on swallowing—see SORE THROAT, pages 91–92

Pain on urination—see URINARY CONDITIONS, page 99

Pain on walking—Pain while walking is most commonly due to a disorder of one or more of the joints and muscles involved. A particular condition, called intermittent claudication, produces intense pain in one or both calves after walking a certain distance or after climbing a certain number of stairs. It often indicates a circulation problem and should be reported to your doctor for further investigation.

PALENESS (PALLOR)

Temporary pallor frequently accompanies fright or shock. Persisting pallor may indicate anemia, and, if it is accompanied by undue fatigue, it should be reported to your doctor.

PALPITATIONS

This feeling of the heart beating rarely indicates disease in the heart or elsewhere. It occurs to most of us during stress or excitement and following exertion. Occasional extra heart beats or thumps and variation of the heart rate with breathing also are normal. At other times, palpitations may arise from undue anxiety, nervousness, or worry, particularly about the possibility of heart disease. Palpitations that appear and disappear abruptly and that accompany a rapid pulse rate (a rate substantially higher than the usual 80 beats a minute) may be an indication of a heart disorder and should be discussed with your doctor. Other common conditions that can cause palpitations are anemia, digestive disorders (especially the night after a binge), or thyroid disease.

You Should See Your Doctor about Palpitations:

Now If your pulse rate is more than 120 beats a minute and you have pain in the chest or shortness of breath.

Within 12 hours If your pulse is persistently irregular or its rate is persistently more than 100 beats a minute.

Within 7 days In all other cases of continuous or repeated attacks of palpitations.

What your doctor may do. He will check your pulse rate and rhythm, measure your blood pressure, and examine your heart and lungs. He may ask you to exercise briskly and then repeat his examinations. He may arrange for an electrocardiogram (ECG) or for further investigations by a heart specialist (cardiologist). He may give you drugs to regulate the heart rate.

What you can do. Don't get into an "I've got heart disease" frame of mind; you probably haven't. Approach the situation as calmly as you can. Deal with anything that might be causing you anxiety or worry.

POISONING

Poisons may be swallowed, inhaled, or absorbed through the skin.

FIRST AID FOR POISONING

If the Patient is Not Conscious

1. If he is not breathing, proceed as on page 32 from Number 4.

2. If he is choking, proceed as on page 31 from Number 1.

3. After these measures have been completed, lay the patient in the recovery position (see page 98).

If the Patient is Conscious

1. Try to find out what poison was taken.

2. If the poison is a *petroleum product or a strong acid or alkali,* move to Number 4 below. *Do not try to make the patient vomit.*

3. For ingestion of any other poison, try to make the patient vomit by agitating the back of his throat with your fingers.

4. Give frequent drinks of plain or salted water or milk to dilute the poison and protect the lining of the stomach.

5. Get an ambulance or doctor. If the patient goes to the hospital, send any information you have about the poison, any remaining poison, or any vomit with him.

6. Keep an eye on the patient all the time you are waiting. He may lapse into unconsciousness or, if suicidal, make another attempt.

If the poisoning has been inhaled: If in an enclosed space, spend a few moments ventilating the room by smashing windows or fanning the air with the door, etc. Drag the victim out into the open air before starting resuscitation (see pages 31–34).

If the poison has been absorbed through the skin after exposure to agricultural or industrial processes: Symptoms of agricultural or industrial poisoning develop gradually; sometimes they do not appear until after exposure to the toxic chemicals has ceased. Warning signs are faintness, sweating, thirst, nausea, vomiting, and stomachache. Remove the patient from the area and make him lie down. Carefully remove contaminated clothes. Wash the affected skin areas with soap and water. Give the patient as much to drink as he can take; plain, salted, or sugared water is best. Be prepared to resuscitate the patient, since breathing may stop suddenly (see pages 31–34).

RASHES

Skin rashes may be due to many causes. They may affect large areas of the body, as in measles or chicken pox, or small areas, as in shingles or dermatitis. Skin disorders can be complicated conditions; so *do not put anything on your skin* except, perhaps, calamine lotion until you have seen your doctor. Whether you should bother your doctor about a rash is a difficult decision to make, but your pharmacist may be able to advise you. Or you may be able to discuss the problem with your doctor over the phone; that way, your doctor can decide whether you should keep an eye on the rash for a day or two or whether special arrangements must be made so you won't pass on an infectious disease to other people.

RHEUMATISM

see *Joint pain and muscle pain,* pages 83–84

"RUN DOWN"

see FATIGUE, page 56

SCALDS

see BURNS, pages 36–38

SHIVERING

see TREMBLING AND TWITCHING, pages 95–96, and TEMPERATURE, pages 94–95

SHOCK

In medical terms, shock is the physical collapse of several vital body systems. It most commonly results from large wounds, extensive bruising, heavy internal or external bleeding, fractures, or burns. A patient in shock becomes cold, clammy, and "deathly" pale; his breathing is rapid, shallow, and almost panting; his pulse rate is weak and rapid (usually over 100 beats a minute compared with the usual 80 beats a minute); and he becomes increasingly mentally disturbed, changing from agitation and restlessness at first to collapse and unconsciousness later. Shock—rather than actual injury—often kills people. It usually develops gradually so you must be constantly on the watch for it. And you must prevent shock if you hope to increase a patient's chances of survival. Prompt and effective first aid measures to prevent shock can make a difference between life and death. Once shock has developed, however, little in the way of first aid can reverse it. Consequently you must be aware of the threat and prevent it. (For electric shock, see ELECTRICAL INJURIES, page 50.)

First Aid to Prevent Shock

1. Stop any severe bleeding (see BLEEDING, pages 25–29).

2. Get the patient into the best position; lay him down on his side with the bottom part of his body propped up so he is lying in a sleeping position but with his head lower than his legs. You may raise the foot end of the board, stretcher, or bed on which the patient has been laid or place a pile of coats, rugs, or blankets under his legs if he is lying on the ground. *Do not* leave a patient sitting slumped in a chair or against a wall or stretched out flat on his back.

3. Loosen tight clothing around the neck, chest, waist, or legs.

4. Keep the patient warm. Cover him with anything available—a coat, rug, or blanket. If he is on the ground, remember to put something underneath him as well as over him. But do not pile too much on top of him; two or three layers usually are enough. And *do not* use hot-water bottles or any form of direct heat.

5. Dress any wounds as necessary (see WOUNDS, pages 104–5 and BURNS, page 36) but do not aggravate any possible fractures. Make the patient as comfortable as possible but *do not* give him anything to eat or drink unless he has severe burns. If he has severe burns, give him water to drink.

6. Stay close to him; he may become restless and roll off whatever you have placed him on. Try to calm him with solid assurances, not vague platitudes. Tell him as much as possible about what has happened, what you are doing step by step, what has happened to his possessions or car, and what has been told to his family. Do not make unguarded remarks

within earshot; he may not be unconscious. And do not whisper in front of the patient; whispering suggests the worst. Get rid of all spectators who are not actually helping.

7. Get an ambulance as quickly as possible. Intensive care, particularly a blood transfusion, may be necessary to save the patient's life.

SLEEPLESSNESS

Sleeping is one of the necessities of life, and interference with it is a common and disturbing complaint. Interference with sleep may involve difficulty getting to sleep, interrupted sleep, or awakening too soon. Worry, tension, and depression are by far the most common causes of sleeplessness, but pain, uncomfortable surroundings, fever, difficulty in breathing while lying down (orthopnea), a need to urinate frequently, and dyspepsia that becomes worse when lying down (as with hiatus hernia), also may give rise to it. Do not try to battle sleeping problems on your own for too long; remember that persistent sleeplessness will cause daytime problems too, such as drowsiness, lack of concentration, and irritability. If you have difficulty in sleeping that continues for more than two weeks, discuss the problem with your doctor.

What your doctor may do. The doctor will try to identify and treat the cause of the problem without prescribing sleeping pills. Sleeping pills are a last resort. They are considered only if other measures have failed. For, although some are less strong than others, all sleeping pills have drawbacks. They reduce alertness during the day and may be addictive.

What you can do. There are many ways in which you can help yourself. The most important is to make sure that there aren't any unresolved tensions left over from the day. If possible, settle all family quarrels before you go to bed; they should not be allowed to hang over into the next day anyway. When you are in bed and before you actually try to go to sleep, go over in your mind all the events of the day from the time you woke up. Things happen to us so fast during the day that we cannot really absorb them all. Things happen too fast for our minds to "digest" them properly. But that "undigested" material may disturb sleep. Quietly reviewing the day's activities not only makes sleep much easier but considerably reduces the build-up of mental indigestion that often turns tension and stress into strain and breakdown.

Quietness, warmth, and a firm mattress also aid sleep, but any gadgets do not. Adequate physical fatigue can be important; it helps if your body is tired as well as your mind. So a 2:00 A.M. walk may successfully deal with insomnia if you don't get much exercise in your job, but daytime exertion is just as effective and much less worrisome. And if you have something going around and around in your head and you can't sleep, spend a half-hour reading Raymond Chandler or Jane Austen or listening to Joan Armatrading or Brahms. It will be less stressful and more effective than tossing and turning.

Regarding sleeping tablets as a last resort. Sleeping tablets may be addictive and they make you less alert, less aware, less alive. Those few regular users of sleeping tablets who have learned to do without them can hardly believe the difference in their enjoyment of life. At times of exceptional stress and upset, sleeping tablets may be needed and should be used. At such times, take an adequate dose to ensure sleep a half-hour before you intend to go to bed on three or five nights. Take half the dose on the next three nights. Then keep the tablets beside your bed but take one only if you are still restless an hour (by your watch) after going to bed.

SORES

see ULCERS, pages 96–97

SORE THROAT

Most sore throats are due to a viral rather than a bacterial infection. They may involve the back of the throat (pharyngitis) or the tonsils (tonsillitis). Soreness of the throat may be accompanied by pain and difficulty swallowing, and the glands under the lower jaw may be swollen and tender. Since sore throats are so common, you should know which are likely to require medical care and which can safely be let alone for a few days.

You Should See Your Doctor about Sore Throat:

Within 12 hours If you have had rheumatic fever or nephritis; if you have a widespread rash; or if your temperature is over 102° F (38.9° C).

Within 24 hours If your tonsils have a white or yellow coating; or if the soreness has lasted for more than two days without improvement.

What your doctor may do. The doctor will examine your throat and perhaps your neck, nose, ears, and chest. He will wipe the back of the throat with a cotton swab and send the material to the laboratory for analysis. If you have had frequent attacks, he may send you to a throat specialist to decide whether you should have your tonsils removed. If your sore throat is due to a bacterial infection, he will prescribe an appropriate antibiotic. Most sore throats are, however, caused by viruses and cannot be treated with antibiotics. He will prescribe other treatment to ease the soreness.

What you can do. Gargle four or five times a day with hot salt water or an aspirin solution. Dissolve two teaspoons of salt or two aspirin tablets into a cup of hot water. Swallow the aspirin solution after gargling. In between gargles, suck some soothing lozenges.

SPLINTERS

What you can do. If the splinter is sticking out from the skin or from under a nail, with tweezers, grip the splinter as close to the skin or nail as possible and pull it out in one movement. If the splinter is completely embedded in the skin, sterilize a large needle by holding the sharp end in a flame for thirty seconds. Use the needlepoint to open the track of the splinter by moving toward the splinter's entry point. Do not move the other way; you may drive the splinter further into the skin. And do not move from the side; you may break the splinter in two. After lifting the splinter out with tweezers, sterilize the wound with antiseptic and keep the wound covered with a dressing for two days.

SPOTS

see RASHES, pages 87–88

SPRAINS

see INJURIES, pages 65–72

SUFFOCATION

see BREATHING, Stopped, pages 31–34

SWALLOWING

Difficulty in swallowing (dysphagia) may be due to obstruction in the esophagus. A foreign body or growth may obstruct the esophagus from the inside, or an enlarged thyroid gland may press on it from the outside. If difficulty in swallowing is accompanied by *pain*, the problem probably is due to inflammation (tonsillitis, pharyngitis, or esophagitis).

What you can do. Gargle with hot salt water or something similar. Report to your doctor any pain or difficulty in swallowing that lasts for more than three days. (See also INDIGESTION, page 63, and SORE THROAT, page 92.)

SWEATING

Abnormal sweating may occur with a fever, the change of life, an overactive thyroid gland, nervousness or anxiety, or simply a group of overactive sweat glands. There is no simple remedy for excessive sweating, but if it persists for more than a week or two, consult your doctor. He will be able to identify and treat the problem.

SWELLING

Swelling of the eye is probably due to inflammation; swelling of the neck, to a thyroid disorder; swelling of the abdomen, to gas, distension of the intestinal tract, fluid in the abdominal cavity (ascites), a distended bladder, or pregnancy; swelling of the scrotum, to inflammation, a tumor in the testicles, or water on the testicles (hydrocele). All require medical attention. (See also LUMPS, page 73.)

TEMPERATURE

Human temperatures that are too low (hypothermia) fall below 95° F (35° C). Low temperatures range from 95° to 97° F (35° to 36° C). Normal temperatures range from 97° to 99° F (36° to 37° C). A slight fever means a temperature between 99° and 101° F (37° and 38° C). A moderate fever is between 101° and 103° F (38° and 39° C). A high temperature falls between 103° and 105° F (39° and 40° C). A dangerously high temperature is above 105° F (40.5° C). A high temperature is almost always due to a generalized infection, such as influenza, or a localized infection, such as tonsillitis or a badly infected wound. It also may be due to heat stroke or, in children, to excitement or excessive crying or screaming. As the temperature rises, the patient often feels cold and may shiver. When it is high, he feels hot, and he may sweat profusely, which tends to bring the temperature down. If the temperature is dangerously high, it may be accompanied by delirium and, particularly in children, by convulsions.

You Should See Your Doctor about a Raised Temperature:

Within 12 hours If an infant's fever has not improved within a day; if a child's fever has not improved within two days; in any patient's fever accompanied by convulsions, delirium, undue drowsiness, an earache, or a severe headache.

Within 24 hours If the fever has not improved within 60 hours or has persisted for more than four days; if the fever is accompanied by any other symptom associated with a particular condition.

What your doctor may do. The doctor will examine you to discover the cause of the high temperature. He may take samples of urine or blood for laboratory analysis. He may—but only rarely—admit you to the hospital for observation, further tests, and nursing care.

What you can do. Remain indoors where the temperature is controlled. Wear light clothing or remain covered only with a single sheet and blanket so your body can cool off. You may not be able to eat for a few days but be sure to drink enough fluid to replace what you are losing in sweat. Drink between three and four pints of liquid a day. You may drink whatever you like as long as it has a reasonably high salt content. Aspirin and acetaminophen will help bring your temperature down. You should take two tablets every four hours. If a patient's temperature rises above 104° F (39.5° C), you may be able to physically cool him off by sponging him with cool (not cold) water in bed or by placing him in a few inches of tepid water in the bathtub and sponging him there. (For a discussion of *low temperature,* see EXPOSURE on page 52.)

TREMBLING AND TWITCHING

Trembling and twitching occur to most of us at times of great excitement or agitation, strenuous exertion, or a rapidly rising temperature. Shaking or tremors in one part of the body may be caused by disorders of the nervous system, such as Parkinson's disease and St. Vitus' dance (chorea), disorders of the thyroid, a habit or a tic. If the condition persists, consult your doctor.

ULCERS

Ulcers are holes in the layer of tissue that covers or lines all parts of the body (epithelium). Ulcers may occur on the skin and are called sores. They also may occur internally in the stomach or part of the intestine (gastric and duodenal ulcers).

Mouth ulcers—are a common and often painful problem. Ulcers on the lips, which are called cold sores (herpes labialis), are caused by a virus. Ulcers inside the mouth may occur after injury to the lining of the mouth from a broken tooth or an accidental bite, or they may occur by themselves (aphtha). More serious causes of ulcers in the mouth, such as cancer and syphilis, are not common; but if you are concerned about a mouth sore or if the ulcer has persisted for more than two weeks, consult your doctor about it.

What you can do. Cold sores and other nonserious mouth sores always heal by themselves in about a week; so there is little you can do about them. Do not touch the sores with your fingers because you could spread the infection to other parts of the body. You may daub the ulcers with an antiseptic-soaked cotton ball to ease the soreness and prevent infection by bacteria in the air. You may spread zinc oxide ointment over the sore every three or four hours.

Other ulcers—Ulcers on other parts of the body may be due to many causes. Varicose veins or "poor circulation" may cause ulcerations on the legs. Infected or poorly healed wounds may develop ulcers. Skin cancer also may produce ulcers.

Ulcers on the genital or anal area should be reported to your doctor, particularly if there was any chance of exposure to syphilis. The ulcer of early syphilis has been described as a single, round, painless sore. However, a great many ulcers that subsequently prove to be caused by syphilis are quite different in character. Since a syphilis ulcer usually will heal by itself in one or two weeks, people believe the sore couldn't have been anything to worry about. In reality, the disappearance of the sore simply marks the end of the first stage of the disease.

What you can do. Sensible home treatment for skin ulcers consists of cleaning the sore with an antiseptic solution, applying an antiseptic cream, and covering the area with a dressing. If the ulcer has not healed in two weeks, consult your doctor. *Do not* try a succession of creams and ointments, hoping to find the best.

UNCONSCIOUSNESS

The possible causes of unconsciousness or coma are many. The common ones include collapse, a head injury, stroke, an overdose of drugs or other types of poisoning, diabetes, and hysteria. The most important task, however, is not to search for the cause but to give immediate first aid. Consider anyone who does not respond to pain as unconscious. Pinch the ear or the back of the heel hard. If there is no reaction, regard the patient as unconscious and promptly begin first aid.

First Aid for Unconsciousness

1. If the patient is breathing move to Step 3. If not, begin resuscitation (see pages 31–34).

2. If there is serious bleeding, stop it (see BLEEDING, pages 25–29). If not, move to Step 3.

3. Look for fractures. Since the patient can't tell you where it hurts, you must look for obvious deformities. Compare the two sides of the body and move your hands carefully, but firmly, over the body. If the patient has fallen from a considerable height, assume that he has sustained fractures, probably of the spine as well as of other parts of the body. If you

suspect the patient has a fractured spine or other serious injuries, *do not* move him. Ensure that his airway is clear by running two fingers around the mouth and back of the throat and be prepared to begin resuscitation if he stops breathing (see pages 31–34).

4. If the patient has no fractures, place him in the *recovery position:*

- Kneel down on the side of the patient toward which you will turn him.
- Put both arms close to the sides of the body.
- Gently turn the patient toward you and over onto his side.
- Pull the upper arm out until it is at a right angle to the body and then bend the elbow.
- Pull up the upper leg so the thigh is at a right angle to the body and the knee is bent.
- Pull the other arm out behind the body so the body is not resting on it.
- Put the head to one side and keep the mouth clear of mucus.

5. Dress any wounds (see WOUNDS, pages 104–5).

6. Keep the patient warm by covering him with a coat or blanket and take any other necessary steps to prevent shock (see SHOCK, pages 88–90).

7. Send for an ambulance and medical help. *Do not* leave the patient alone; he may suddenly need further help, such as resuscitation. *Do not* attempt to give the patient food or drink of any kind.

8. Look for any clues to the cause of unconsciousness—an accident, an empty drug bottle, or a medical warning bracelet or card in the patient's wallet, purse, or pocket.

9. If you are able, keep a record of the patient's breathing and pulse rates and the size of his pupils every fifteen minutes.

URETHRAL DISCHARGE

Discharge and pain, usually on urination (dysuria), are almost always an indication of a sexually transmitted or venereal disease, and these symptoms must be reported to your doctor for expert assessment and treatment. He may refer you to a venereal disease clinic or to a specialist.

URINARY CONDITIONS

Pain on urination (dysuria), increased frequency of urination, and blood-stained urine (hematuria) are most commonly caused by an infection in the urinary tract. Frequent urination may be associated with such conditions as diabetes or a kidney disorder, or it may be an indication of pregnancy in women and enlargement of the prostate gland in men. Needing to get up at night to urinate (nocturia), needing to go in a hurry, or difficulty in beginning or in going at all also are often associated with prostatic enlargement. For any urinary abnormality that persists for more than a few days or returns repeatedly, consult your doctor.

You Should See Your Doctor about a Urinary Condition:

Within 12 hours If there is discharge from the penis; or if the urine is bloody.

Within 24 hours If there is fever, back or abdominal pain, or vomiting; or if pain on urination has persisted for more than two days.

Within 7 days In all other cases of difficult urination or abnormal urine.

What your doctor may do. The doctor will examine your abdomen and genital organs. If he examines the prostate gland, he will probe the area through the rectum. He may take a specimen of the discharge or the urine for laboratory analysis. He may conduct some preliminary tests on the urine in the office, order further investigations involving blood tests or an X-ray of the urinary tract (intravenous pyelogram), or refer you to a specialist. If the problem is a urinary infection, the doctor will prescribe an appropriate antibiotic.

What you can do. Drink plenty of fluids, about a half-pint every half-hour during the day. If your symptoms persist for more than two days, see your doctor. Don't urinate for a few hours before you see him because he probably will want a fresh specimen.

VAGINAL CONDITIONS

Vaginal discharge is a common and widely misunderstood condition. The amount of discharge varies from one woman to another and may increase in certain situations, particularly those related to sexual matters. What is important is not the amount but the type of discharge. Clear, mucous discharge is probably not due to disease. Discharge that is discolored, is accompanied by soreness or irritation of the vagina or vaginal lips (vulva), or is smelly may be related to infection in the genital organs. Thin, yellow discharge indicates infection from Trichomonas; thick, white discharge indicates thrush; and brown discharge indicates internal bleeding. Internal bleeding may be due to erosion or ulceration of the neck of the womb or cervix or to cancer of the womb. It must, therefore, be thoroughly investigated, especially when it occurs in women between the ages of 40 and 60. Contrary to general belief, gonorrhea in women does not usually cause vaginal discharge or any other symptom. (See also MENSTRUAL PROBLEMS, pages 73–74, and *Pain on intercourse*, page 83.)

You Should See Your Doctor about a Vaginal Discharge:

Within 12 hours If it is accompanied by a fever or abdominal pain; or if there is a possibility of exposure to venereal disease.

Within 24 hours If it is blood-stained or brown and you are not expecting a period soon; or if it is smelly or accompanied by pain on urination, soreness, or irritation.

Within 7 days In all other cases of worrisome discharge.

What your doctor may do. The doctor will ask about the character of the discharge and about recent sexual contact. He will examine the vagina with a gloved hand and with a plastic or metal instrument (vaginal speculum). (The procedure is unpleasant but not usually painful.) He will take specimens from the vagina and the neck of the womb and perhaps from the urethra and rectum for laboratory analysis. If the cause of the problem is straightforward, the doctor will prescribe tablets to be taken by mouth, medicine to be inserted into the vagina, or cream to be used in the vagina or on its lips.

What you can do. Maintain good vaginal hygiene. Wash or bathe before and after you make love. Vaginal douching is *not* advised. Douching may wash infection further into the womb. Because tight-fitting jeans, tights, tampons, and vaginal deodorants cause vaginal discharge in some women, they may have to be avoided. Do not let an unpleasant discharge continue for more than a week before consulting your doctor.

VOMITING

Vomiting usually is due to irritation or inflammation of the inside of the stomach or to stimulation of the vomiting reflex at the back of the throat. Common causes of vomiting are eating too much, drinking too much alcohol, eating or drinking impure food or water, an infection of the stomach, a peptic ulcer, stomach cancer, gall bladder disease, early pregnancy, travel sickness, migraine headaches, stress, and severe pain. (See also INDIGESTION, pages 62–64.)

You Should See Your Doctor about Vomiting:

Now If the vomit consists of pure blood or is heavily blood-stained or black or looks like coffee grounds; if it is accompanied by intense, persistent abdominal pain; if it follows a recent head injury.

Within 12 hours If you have black or tar-like stools or bring up anything unexpectedly; or if it is accompanied by a severe headache or dizziness.

Within 24 hours If it is frequent; if it is accompanied by abdominal pain other than indigestion; or if you feel very ill.

Within 7 days If it is persistent or recurs; or if you may be pregnant.

What your doctor may do. The doctor will examine your abdomen. If the cause of vomiting is straightforward, he will prescribe medicine, give dietary advice, and arrange to see you again if the trouble persists. If vomiting persists, he may arrange for an X-ray of the stomach (barium swallow) or gall bladder (cholecystogram), or he may refer you to a specialist. If you have any bleeding in the stomach, he may admit you to the hospital.

What you can do. Do *not* take solid foods which will make you vomit more. Do sip bland fluids—water or milk, not fizzy or alcoholic drinks—to replace what you are losing in the vomit. Milk or a teaspoon of bicarbonate of soda dissolved in a cup of water may be helpful. After vomiting is over, take a day or two to work up to your usual diet.

WEAKNESS

Weakness may affect the body as a whole (see FATIGUE, page 56) or a part of the body when muscular strength diminishes or disappears completely (paralysis). Weakness in one part of the body may follow a stroke or be due to high blood pressure, a disorder of the nervous or muscular systems, or an emotional disturbance, such as hysteria. Weakness may be the first indication of a serious underlying condition.

You Should See Your Doctor about Weakness:

Within 24 hours In all cases.

WEIGHT

Loss of—Definite and persistent weight loss should be taken seriously. It sometimes is the only indication of such serious underlying diseases as cancer, diabetes, a thyroid disorder, or tuberculosis. Common indications of persistent weight loss are a thinner appearance or loose-fitting clothes. Check for weight loss by weighing yourself once a week on the same scale in similar clothes and at the same time of day. If you are continually losing weight, see your doctor within a week or two. Don't delay your trip to the doctor for months while you try to put on weight.

What you can do. Try to stimulate your appetite by taking an *aperitif* a half-hour before you plan to eat. Try to eat more frequent and larger meals, increase the amount of starchy foods—bread, cereals, rice and pasta, potatoes and rich desserts—and get plenty of fresh air and exercise. (See also APPETITE, Too little, pages 21–22.)

Too much—see APPETITE, Too much, page 23

WHEEZING

Wheezing usually means there is some hindrance to normal breathing, such as a narrowing or spasm of the air passages or a partial blockage of the airway due to phlegm (sputum). Wheezing often is accompanied by shortness of breath, and it commonly is associated with asthma, chronic bronchitis, and chest infections. Wheezing that occurs for the first time and lasts for several hours must be investigated by your doctor.

What your doctor may do. The doctor will examine your chest and perhaps order a chest X-ray. He may send you to the hospital or to a chest clinic for further investigation.

What you can do. Home treatment can do little to relieve wheezing. Inhalations of menthol or eucalyptus are sometimes helpful, however (see pages 10–11).

WOUNDS

Wounds range from a small graze (abrasion) to a large open wound (laceration). Although often small, puncture wounds, such as those caused by stabbing or firearms, may penetrate deeply into the body and damage internal structures or carry infection far inside the body. They always should be seen by a doctor. Wounds that have been heavily contaminated by dirt or have been caused by an animal bite also should be seen by a doctor. Other small wounds usually can be treated without medical attention as long as they have not become infected. Large wounds probably need stitching to hold the edges together so healing can occur and scarring can be avoided. Deciding which wounds need stitching and which do not may be difficult. In general, wounds whose edges gape apart, those that are more than an inch long, and wounds from which bleeding is persistent probably should be stitched. If in doubt, get medical advice. (See also INJURIES, pages 65–72; BLEEDING, pages 25–29; BURNS, pages 36–38; BITES AND STINGS, pages 22–25; BRUISING, page 36; and *Wounds to the eye,* page 55.)

First Aid for Wounds

1. If there is severe bleeding, see BLEEDING, pages 25–29.
2. Get the patient to sit or lie down.
3. Remove all clothing around the wound. Tear or cut it away if necessary.
4. Lay a piece of clean material or a dressing lightly across the wound to protect it from contamination while you are getting things ready.
5. Assemble everything you are likely to need.
6. Wash your hands as thoroughly as possible. Scrub them for two minutes with soap and water if you can.
7. Remove any loose objects or material from the wound with tweezers or with your fingers. Brush any dirt or gravel away with a clean handkerchief or a piece of gauze. *Do not* poke inside the wound. *Do not* attempt to remove anything

embedded in the wound. Things embedded in a wound probably have done all the damage they are going to do and pulling them out may make matters worse. *Do not* disturb blood clots; you may make the wound start bleeding again.

8. Wash a wide area of skin around the injury, using soap and water or an antiseptic on a cotton ball or gauze swab. Do not touch the wound itself. Continue cleaning the area methodically in a series of separate strokes. Start each stroke close to the wound and wipe away from the wound.

9. You can now clean the wound itself. Using balls of cotton gauze swabs, flush water or a mild antiseptic into the wound. *Do not* rub or wipe the wound. Let the antiseptic dry before dressing the wound.

10. Dress the wound. Usually dry dressings are preferable to the use of antiseptic creams. Since moisture promotes infection and hampers the repair processes, try to keep the wound as dry as possible. In general, do not cover wounds with totally enclosing adhesive dressings. They tend to build up moisture and keep the wound from drying. Remove the dressing and leave the wound open to the air as soon as it has stopped oozing.

For covering wounds, prepared sterile dressings are ideal. Next in preference is a layer of clean gauze that is large enough to amply cover the wound and is topped with a thick wad of cotton. If neither of these is available, use any clean cloth—a handkerchief, napkin, or towel—taking care not to handle the side that will be placed next to the wound. If an object is sticking out of the wound, make sure that your dressing does not force it in further. Instead build a protective pad around the object. The bandage holding your dressing in place should not be too tight, but it must be firm enough so the dressing will not slip off (see pages 109–10). In an emergency, a scarf, necktie, stockings, or tights make adequate bandages. When appropriate, rest the wounded part of the body in a sling.

11. Remember to watch for the development of shock and be prepared to prevent it (see SHOCK, pages 88–90).

6.

Home Nursing Care

You will find advice about how to treat particular symptoms and what procedures to follow in emergency situations on pages 19–105. You should have a medicine chest with all the equipment you need to handle emergencies and minor medical problems. (A list of the contents of most home medicine chests is given on page 8.) You also should know how to provide general nursing care at home.

GENERAL NURSING CARE

Get into the habit of keeping a watchful eye on anybody that you are nursing or looking after. Notice the patient's color, degree of sweating, facial expression, and state of mind. Occasionally changes in temperature and pulse rate may be important; so you should know how to take them. Generally, however, your estimate of whether somebody is ill or not is a better guide to their need for medical attention than the thermometer. And remember that 98.6° F (36.9° C) is not a magic figure and that any variation from this temperature does not necessarily mean illness. The 98.6° F temperature is an average, and wide variations on either side of it—certainly from 97° F (36.1° C) to 99° F (37.4° C)—are not unusual (see TEMPERATURE, pages 94–95).

To take a person's temperature. Shake the mercury down by holding the top of the thermometer between your finger and thumb and by jerking your hand violently up and down from the wrist. Stand clear of any furniture or other obstacles. Place the bulb of the thermometer under the patient's tongue for two minutes; have the patient firmly close the lips but not bite on the thermometer. Or place the thermometer in the armpit for three minutes; have the patient hold the arm firmly against his side. Remove the thermometer and, holding it level with your eyes, slowly turn it between your fingers until the mercury line appears. The end of the line of mercury corresponds to the patient's temperature and can be compared with the "normal" temperature, which is usually marked by an arrow. Shake down the mercury and wash the thermometer before putting it away.

To take the pulse rate. Put the tips of the middle three fingers of the left hand just above the heel of the right thumb (see Appendix, page 213, for an illustration). Move them around gently until you feel a slow pulsation. Using a watch with a second hand, count the pulsations for a quarter of a minute and multiply the result by four to get the pulse rate. The normal rate in adults is between 70 and 80 beats a minute, but it is much higher in infants—up to 140 beats a minute—or after exertion.

Care of wounds, inflammation, and minor injuries. The basic aim is to prevent infection and promote healing and recovery. Antiseptics stop germs from breeding but often are not strong enough to kill them. Disinfectants kill germs, if given time to do so, but they usually are too strong to use on the body. They damage healthy tissue and interfere with the healing process as well. There are several good antiseptics available. Chlorhexidine Hibiclens is effective and safe.

When dressing wounds, grazes, bites, boils, etc., keep the

risk of infection to a minimum by following as closely as you can the techniques that are used in hospitals. Keep everything as sterile as possible. Wear a mask to prevent germs in your nose and mouth from getting into the wound. Sterilize instruments by boiling them for ten minutes immediately before use. Make sure that the water completely covers the instruments. Do not touch the instruments after they have been sterilized unless your hands have been scrubbed with soap and hot water for at least five minutes. Take care that you have made all your preparations and removed any soiled dressings before you scrub your hands; all your efforts will be in vain if you touch something that is unsterile. Pour a small quantity of an antiseptic solution into a bowl beforehand so you do not have to touch the bottle. Ask an assistant to get a dressing from a fresh and preferably sterilized pack and to tear open the wrapping without touching the contents. Use each piece of cotton or gauze only once and then throw it away. To clean the wound, work systematically, using light but deliberate and overlapping strokes that sweep outward from the center of the wound.

When the wound is clean, apply a dressing, taking care not to touch the part of the dressing that will be placed on the wound itself. Gauze makes the best dressing, but the clean inner side of a handkerchief or napkin may be used in an emergency. By applying a hot iron to the handkerchief or napkin just before use, you can kill off many germs. You may add padding of cotton socks or small towels to protect the wound. To keep the dressing firmly in place, use strips of adhesive or an adhesive bandage. You also may use a sterile dressing that consists of a cotton pad covered by plain gauze and stitched to a bandage.

Bandages, although not used as much as they used to be, still often must be placed on minor wounds. Bandaging keeps wound dressings in position and helps provide support and rest to a part of the body that has been strained or sprained (see pages 65–67). Bandages that can exert pressure, such as those made from elastic, are particularly useful for strained or sprained muscles as long as they are not put on too tightly.

When bandaging, stand in front of the patient and make sure that the limb is in the right position before you begin. Work with the bandage held upward, and work upward from below and from the inside out. To make sure the bandage does not slip, make a couple of very firm turns at first. Wrap the rest of the bandage evenly. With each turn, cover two-thirds of the previous one. But take care, especially with bandages containing stretch materials such as elastic, that you do not pull too tightly. Tight-fitting bandages may interfere with the circulation and cause swelling, discoloration, or a pins-and-needles sensation.

A cold compress immediately applied to the site of an injury may limit the amount of swelling and bruising that develops. A dressing, handkerchief, or napkin should be thoroughly soaked in cold but not icy water, wrung out until dripping stops, and loosely bandaged onto the injured part. As soon as the dressing begins to dry or becomes warm, remove it and repeat the process.

Home physical therapy. Many strains (see page 66) and rheumatic conditions can be helped considerably by simple home physical therapy. In fact, your doctor may recommend such treatment for certain conditions. If you are in doubt about whether your condition will benefit from home physical therapy, ask your doctor about it before you start.

In the acute stage, usually immediately after injury, an inflamed part of the body needs rest more than anything else. But heat is also useful. It increases the blood supply to the area and makes the affected part less painful to move. In the care of inflammations such as boils (see page 30), heat usually is applied in a hot compress or poultice. To treat injured or inflamed muscles, ligaments, or joints, heat is best given via a heat lamp, hot-water bottle, or small space heater. If sensibly used, a small space heater can do almost as much good as an expensive heat lamp. Put the space heater on a table and sit in front of it, with the affected part uncovered and not less than three feet away from the heat, for about fifteen minutes three or four times a day. You should be close enough to feel the heat but not close enough to burn your skin.

Unless there is severe inflammation, the heat treatment should be followed by massage. A massage can be more effective if the skin is oily, but it's the massage that counts, not what you rub on; so you may as well use something safe and inexpensive like liniment. When giving a massage, remember that gentle rubbing will not do much good; what is required is a steady kneading movement. Get the balls of the thumbs well into the affected area and rub the skin and muscles for ten to fifteen minutes.

As the condition improves, gradually increase exercise until you regain normal activity. You should do neither too much nor too little, and you should be able to gauge your activity level for yourself. As soon as possible, try to put the injured part of the body through its normal range of movements. Beyond a certain point, pain probably will make some of these movements difficult or impossible. Exercise up to but not beyond this point from six to twelve times in each exercise session. On each occasion, hold the affected part in position for ten seconds. Have an exercise session every hour while you are away from work.

Obtaining Medical Help

If you must get a message to your doctor, the ambulance service, or the police, make sure that it is accurate, complete, and brief. Say only what the patient has noticed, not what you think may be the cause. For instance, report that the patient complained of a terrible pain in the chest and then collapsed. Do not say that he has had a heart attack. You may waste valuable time if the doctor has to cross-examine you unnecessarily about exactly what you mean. Do not, in the heat of the moment, forget to mention important facts. Give the patient's full name and age and include directions for finding or recognizing your house or apartment building as well as the address. Especially at night, have somebody outside to show the way or have the front lights blazing. Don't, in your anxiety, get your doctor involved in a complicated conversation about what might be wrong or how serious the problem might be. The time would be better spent by letting the doctor get on his way to meet the patient. And keep a record, preferably a written one, of the changes in the patient's condition and the home treatment or first aid that has been given. The doctor may find such information helpful.

CARE OF A PATIENT IN BED

People should not be encouraged to stay in bed for more than a day or two unless the doctor has advised it, they have a temperature of over 101° F (38° C), or they feel too ill to get up. Prolonged bedrest can have serious ill effects, particularly in elderly patients. Rest in an armchair after periodic strolls around the room generally is much better. Nevertheless, there are times when people must be confined to bed. And their bedding from the mattress (preferably a firm one) upward should consist of:

- An under blanket.
- An under sheet.
- A piece of plastic sheeting where the patient's buttocks will rest if he is likely to wet the bed.
- A sheet placed on the bed where the patient's trunk and waist will rest and tucked in so most of it is on one side. (This "drawsheet" is intended to be pulled across a little at a time every few hours so the patient can lie on a fresh sheet but you don't have to change the whole sheet.)
- A top sheet.
- One or two top blankets and a quilt or comforter, depending on the temperature in the room.
- Pillows according to the doctor's orders and the patient's comfort.

The bedclothes should stay firmly in place, but they should

not be too tight or smothering. The bed should be warmed beforehand by means of an electric blanket or hot-water bottle, but the blanket should be switched off or the bottle should be removed before the patient gets into bed.

If possible, the patient should get out of bed and sit on a chair while his bed is remade. If he is too ill to get out of bed, you will have to make the bed with a patient in it. You may need an assistant, and you should have two chairs—one on which to place the clean bedclothes and one at the foot of the bed.

To make a bed with the patient in it:

- Remove the quilt or comforter and loosen the bedclothes all around the bed.
- If there is a coverlet, fold it back on itself, take it off the bed, and lay it across the chair at the foot of the bed.
- If there are two blankets, repeat this process with the top one.
- Ease out the top sheet but leave the patient covered with the second blanket.
- Standing on the side of the bed with the short end of the drawsheet, roll the patient toward you. Take care to fully support the patient so he cannot slip off the bed.
- Roll the drawsheet, plastic sheeting, under sheet, and under blanket toward the patient so they lie in a tight roll behind him.
- Roll the patient onto his other side so the old bedding can be removed later.
- Place the clean bedclothes, with the farthest half rolled up, at the patient's back. Spread the nearest half across the bed and tuck it in tightly so there are no creases.
- Roll the patient back onto his other side and across the two rolls of bedding.
- Remove the old bedding and spread out the farthest half of the new bedding, tucking it in tightly so there are no creases.
- Place a clean top sheet across the patient.

- Ease out the top blanket that has been covering the patient and place it on top of the sheet.
- Straighten out and tuck in the bedding all around; if necessary, pull the mattress up to the head of the bed.
- Replace the second blanket, coverlet, and quilt.

Comfort in Bed. Few people like to be confined to bed. Unless too ill to care, people feel restricted, isolated, uncomfortable, and depressed. A major part of successful nursing care is understanding these feelings, however unreasonable they may be, and counteracting them.

To make a patient more comfortable, you may change the patient's position.

- To give the patient complete rest and care for spinal conditions such as a slipped disk, place the patient in the recumbent position—flat on his back with only one pillow.
- An alternative position for complete rest or care of painful conditions of the back or buttocks, is the prone position— flat on his belly with his head on one side.
- Another alternative position for complete rest and for those who are unconscious is the "recovery" or semiprone position—on one side.
- The patient who is improving and wishes to sit up may be supported with three or four pillows in a half-sitting (or semirecumbent) position.
- Patients who are getting better or who have difficulty in breathing when lying down may be placed in an upright sitting or "convalescent" position.

For a patient who can sit up in bed, the periodic collapse of the pillows behind him can be annoying. So try to borrow from a local hospital or improvise a firm, secure back rest. And put a pillow at the foot of the bed to keep the patient from slipping down. A patient frequently feels cut off and "forgotten" in the bedroom. Try to drop in and see how he is from time to time. And set up a reliable way for him to call you; have him use a handbell, gong, or even a stick with which to bang on the floor. Make sure that the patient has all the things that he may want—a drink, makeup, newspapers, books, or a radio—close at hand. If he is unable to get out of bed to go to the bathroom, you will need to make arrangements for a bedpan or urinal.

An important part of making the patient comfortable involves keeping him clean and fresh. If he is not able to get to the bathroom, he should have a daily bed bath. To give a bed bath, you need a bowl of warm water, a large jug of hot water, soap, and a washcloth, plus a pail for slops, towels, and clean nightclothes. Change the water whenever it gets cold or too dirty. If the patient finds the powder refreshing, dust on talc after drying each part. To give a bed bath, proceed as follows:

- Remove the top bedclothes and place towels or old blankets on top of and underneath the patient.
- Remove the patient's nightclothes but keep him covered with a towel or blanket.
- Using a washcloth and small towel, wash with soap and water, rinse off, and dry the face, neck, and ears.
- While keeping the rest of the body covered, wash, rinse, and dry one arm from the armpit to the fingers.
- Repeat the process for the other arm.
- Fold the cover up so it lies above the patient's waist, then wash the lower abdomen and genital area. Replace the cover.
- Uncover one leg and wash, rinse, and dry it from the groin down to the toes.
- Repeat the process for the other leg.
- Turn the patient toward you and wash his back from neck to buttocks.
- Put on clean nightclothes and remake the bed.

Remember to pay attention to the patient's hair and nails. If the patient must stay in bed for more than a few days, you must take special care to prevent pressure or bed sores. Bed sores occur on parts of the body that press on the bed; the buttocks, bottom of the back, shoulders, heels, elbows, and hips are at greatest risk. In the prevention of bed sores, the most important points are to keep the bedding and the patient dry and clean. Moisture greatly increases the chance of developing bed sores. Change bedclothes or nightclothes at once if they become soiled. Also keep the sheet under the patient as smooth as possible. Pull the drawsheet through every two or three hours and brush it free of crumbs. At the same time, make sure that the patient moves into a different position. Remove pressure from vulnerable areas as much as possible by using pillows or improvised pads.

Getting a patient in and out of his clothes and in and out of bed requires special care. When helping a patient with a disabled arm or leg to undress, free the sound arm or leg from the clothing first. You then can gently draw the clothes over the damaged limb without hurting it. When helping with dressing, draw the clothes onto the disabled limb first.

When completely undressing somebody who is too ill to help themselves, sit him or her on the edge of the bed and get an assistant to help support him. First remove the shoes and socks; then take the upper clothes off first and put on the top part of the nightclothes. Gently lay the patient back to take off the lower clothes and put on the bottom part of the nightclothes.

When helping a patient out of bed, first put on his dressing gown, then fold the bedclothes down to the bottom of the bed. Lift the patient's legs over the side of the bed as he sits up, put on his socks and slippers, and help him to his feet. Support him carefully while he moves to a chair. Make sure there is nothing on the floor that may trip him. Once the patient is in the chair, wrap a blanket around him, put a pillow behind his head, place a footstool under his feet if he wants one, and make sure that everything he needs is within reach.

CARE OF A SICK CHILD

Should I send for the doctor or not? There are not as many problems in looking after children as many people, especially first-time parents, think. In general, the most reliable guidelines are to follow your common sense and the child's reactions. Your common sense and the child's reaction will not help you in some situations, however. In these situations, you will be uncertain or worried about what is wrong with your child, about its seriousness, and about what to do. If this is the case, consult your doctor. The doctor may not have to see the child at home or at the office. All that may be needed is a telephone conversation with your doctor, in which you describe your child's condition and your worries about him and in which the doctor obtains any other necessary information. The doctor can then decide whether to give you advice over the telephone or to make plans to see and examine the patient. Some medical problems, particularly in babies, require medical attention. Babies often are not able to cope with illness, cannot let you know what feels wrong, and may develop serious disorders in a matter of hours. Advice about the assessment of particular complaints is given under the appropriate heading in the chapter that begins on page 19. But as a general rule, consult your doctor about any child who remains ill, cannot eat, is feverish, is vomiting or has diarrhea, or is reluctant to get out of bed or go to school for more than two days in succession.

Is he really ill or not? All symptoms can be emotional rather than physical in origin, and to decide whether a child is really ill or not is sometimes difficult for the doctor let alone for you. The best advice is to accept the child's version of the situation at least for a day or two. After a day or two to themselves, many children get over their troubles on their own. Urging children to explain why they are reluctant to go to school usually does more harm than good. The fact that a child doesn't want to go to school or wants to stay in bed means that something is wrong. As long as he is not seriously ill, it really doesn't matter whether his temporary upset is physical or emotional in origin. If the problem continues for more than two or three days with no sign of improvement or if there has been a succession of mysterious "illnesses," talk to your doctor.

Should I keep him in bed or not? In general, don't keep a child in bed unless he wants to be there. Even if he has a fever, the child is the best judge of whether he is sick enough to stay in bed. Unless a child is very ill, keeping him away from the family can make him lonely and depressed. It is more likely to hinder recovery than to help. The child does need to be in a fairly constant temperature. So the living room, under blankets on the sofa, with the distractions of the family and the television, is probably the best place for him. But put him to bed early so he can get the extra sleep he may need to deal with his illness. The same rule applies to getting the child up and back to school after a spell in bed. He'll let you know when he doesn't want to stay in bed any longer. In all but a few illnesses, the chance that a child will "overdo things" is small.

What should I give him to eat? If the child feels like eating, let him. If he doesn't, don't force him. Your doctor will tell you if any special dietary rules should be followed. But do make sure that the child is getting plenty to drink. And don't worry if he doesn't have his bowels open for a few days.

Are there any special rules? If there is anything that you must do or not do to treat your child's illness, your doctor will tell you. Remember that a sick child may be irritable and "difficult," and you will have to be patient and give him extra attention, and reassurance. An illness, even if it is not serious, is a big event in a child's life, and the memory of things connected with it often plays a significant part in his emotional development. So you must retain his trust through the first hazards in his life. Tell him as much as you can about his illness; children often are capable of understanding a great deal more than we give them credit for, and their fear of the unknown or the misunderstood usually is greater than their apprehension about something they know will be unpleasant. Certainly don't lie to your child. If he asks, tell him that injections hurt for a moment or two or that the medicine may taste bad, but at the same time, avoid alarming him with any fears that you may have. Above all, give your sick child tender loving care.

PEOPLE WHO NEED SPECIAL CARE

Care of a patient in a cast. The plaster will take about two days to harden. During that time, it must not be subjected to pressure, and the affected part of the body must be kept at rest so the shape of the cast is not distorted. If parts of the body beyond the cast, usually the fingers or toes, become swollen or discolored or produce a persistent "pins-and-needles" sensation or if the part in the cast gets more rather than less uncomfortable, see your doctor as soon as possible. Do not let the cast get wet by washing or being out in the rain. It may get soft. If the plaster becomes soft or is damaged, get the cast repaired as soon as possible. Make sure that you know how much you are allowed to use the damaged part and do not overuse it. When the damaged part is not in use, make sure that the cast is propped up. Place the leg on a stool or chair or put an arm in a sling or on the arm of a chair to reduce the chance of serious swelling inside the cast.

Care of a patient after an operation or childbirth. People are sent home from the hospital after an operation or after childbirth much sooner nowadays than they used to be. Nonetheless, hospitals do not let patients go home until it is safe to do so. When you take a patient home from the hospital, be sure to get as much information as you can about how he should be cared for, including any special requirements for medicine, diet, etc. Having a relative or friend stay in the patient's home or at least call several times a day is a great help during this period. The patient's progress after an operation or childbirth is usually steady and uneventful. But if you have any cause for worry, do not hesitate to talk to your doctor.

Care of a patient after a heart attack. Home treatment of a patient after a heart attack follows the same lines as those given above. You should know how much rest and how much and what kind of activity the hospital doctors want the patient to have. You should know how the doctors plan for the patient to increase his activity.

Care of a patient who has had a colostomy or ileostomy. Surgeons treat some intestinal conditions by making an opening through the wall of the lower abdomen through which the colon or ileum releases waste matter. A disposable bag on a waistband is attached to the opening in the colon (colostomy) or ileum (ileostomy) to collect the material. Many people lead active and full lives after a colostomy or ileostomy. Such surgery sometimes, however, is not easy for patients or their families to come to terms with physically or emotionally, and considerable courage and determination often are required. Detailed advice and supervision are given by the doctor while the patient is in the hospital and afterward. Additional help is available from organizations of people who have had a colostomy or ileostomy and are familiar with the problems that can arise.

Care of a mentally ill person. The kind of care that most likely will help a person who is emotionally disturbed or mentally ill is described on page 51. Detailed needs and patterns of management vary from person to person and with the particular type of illness. Understanding the patient's difficulties and tolerating his shortcomings may be called for in large measure. Most mentally ill patients can exercise some control and take some responsibility for their behavior; so reasoned firmness and the refusal to allow patients to manipulate situations to their own advantage have a place in their care. The continuous care of a mentally ill person can be extremely exhausting. Demanding care of this sort should be shared by as many people as possible. If you have difficulty getting help from others, consult your doctor or your local mental health agency. Make sure that you get away from the care of the patient for at least two two-week periods a year and one weekend every month. If the patient's condition becomes worse and you cannot cope, you must seek help. Nobody likes the idea of sending a friend or family member to a hospital. However, a stubborn refusal to admit "defeat" may not be in the best interests of the patient.

Care of a chronically ill or disabled person. Specific care depends on the illness or disability, but general nursing principles are the same regardless of the problem. For instance, you should encourage the patient to do as much as he can himself, even if he takes longer to do it than you would. For his self-respect, he must maintain whatever independence he can. Also one day he may no longer have your help and should not lose any skill because of disuse. In the care of the disabled, there is no place for unnecessary fussing, but help should not be so frugal that the patient's life is little more than a succession of endurance tests. Remember that many disabled people vary widely in what they are able to do on their good days and on their bad days.

For most disabled people who were previously active in body and mind, the perpetual frustrations of their limited activities and the knowledge that the situation is permanent inevitably lead to periods of intense depression and despair. These periods should be accepted without embarrassment or recrimination. Quiet, patient support is most helpful at such times. A periodic explosion to "let off steam," or an outburst of weeping or cursing at the hand fate has dealt is understandable and is preferable to bottling up the anger and resentment.

The patient's inescapable limitations may be overlaid with needless secondary limitations that spring from the despair and hopelessness which overwhelm the patient when he first becomes disabled. A "settling-down" period during which the patient assesses the "meaning" of his disability in relation to his previous life and during which he tries to come to terms with his disability obviously is necessary. In the "settling-down" period, the patient will be in shock and will be inactive. The inactivity should not go on for too long before the patient makes a start on rehabilitation and resettlement and decides what changes must be made in the pattern of his life. As soon as possible, the patient should make three lists: first, of the things that he cannot do; second, of the things that he can do with difficulty; and third, of the things that he can do without difficulty. Within this framework, the patient must try to construct a completely new life; he must not consider his new life as an incomplete continuation of the life that is now past. Then he must develop a daily timetable so time neither drifts by aimlessly nor hangs heavily on his mind. Despair and boredom are the enemies of the disabled. Filling the timetable with activities is therefore more important than deciding what those activities should be.

The continual care of a chronically ill or disabled person can be physically and mentally exhausting. Get all the help you can and share the work as much as possible among other members of the family or with friends. If you are to give your best, you must get away from the situation periodically. Get away for a least two two-week periods a year and one week-end every month.

Care of a person who is dying. Most of us, even if we are suffering considerably, are unwilling and afraid to die. And none of us can contemplate dying away from our loved ones or in pain with anything but horror. A person should be allowed to die in the familiar, loved, and comfortable surroundings of his home, and he should be cared for by his family, unless there are very strong reasons for hospital care. Terminal care in a hospital, no matter how understanding and efficient the staff may be, is seldom a desirable substitute.

Deciding whether a person should be told that he is dying is extremely difficult. Certainly a person who has not asked directly if he is dying should not have the knowledge forced upon him; the total withdrawal of hope inevitably casts premature and unnecessary darkness over a person's last days. On the other hand, constantly refusing to discuss the subject or giving evasive answers is not helpful either; the patient frequently feels that the situation is worse or that the end is closer than it really is, and he believes he can no longer trust those around him or talk to them openly. In addition, people have the right to know what is going to happen to them because they may have unfinished business that they want to complete.

In reality, most patients do not ask if they are dying. Some prefer to let matters take their course without directly facing the possibility of death. Others know that death has become a probability but see no point and have no need to discuss it. Others ask directly and keep on asking until they get a direct answer. These patients should not be put off by saying that "nobody can be sure" or that "there's always room for hope." They should not be told bluntly, "Yes, you are going to die." They should be told that death is a definite possibility but that there is no certainty about it and no indication of when it might be. Then they should be asked if there are any special things they would like to do to prepare for it.

Once a patient has reached an unspoken understanding or an open acceptance of the possibility or probability of death, he must live life as normally as circumstances permit. The vital features are freedom from pain and an atmosphere of tranquility. With the drugs that are available nowadays, there is no need for anybody to suffer great physical pain. Painkilling drugs should be given regularly so the next dose begins to act before the last has worn off. Painkillers should not be withheld until pain has become severe; the aim should be to keep a step ahead of the pain. As greater pain develops, the dose and the frequency of administration of the drugs probably will have to be increased. Do not hesitate to do so; keeping the patient free from pain far outweighs the possibility of giving too much medication. If the drugs are no longer effectively controlling the pain, tell your doctor as soon as possible. There are many ways in which he can remedy the situation.

The normal household routine should be followed, and the

patient should continue his usual responsibilities as long as possible. He should be encouraged to live fully but on a day-to-day basis. He should have easy access to favorite books, music, food and drink, and people. "Parting" and other emotional, upsetting subjects should be avoided, but business affairs, wills, and possibly unpleasant confidences about events in the patient's past should be discussed. Finally, you must prepare yourself for the bereavement that is to come.

Care of a bereaved person. The death of a loved one, even if it has been expected and is a "merciful release," has intense impact. There is the emptiness and the longing; there are, however undeservedly, feelings of guilt and regret about things that might have been managed differently; often there are practical problems about home or money. Somebody who can share, or at least understand, these burdens is a great help.

The first task after somebody dies is to complete the necessary formalities. The patient's doctor must be informed at once if death was sudden. You can wait until office hours the next day if death was expected. If death was due to an accident or any suspicious circumstances, the police must be informed. In such cases, neither the body nor anything in the room must be touched. In other cases, the undertaker of your choice should be contacted to make arrangements for burial services. To avoid misunderstandings, somebody in the family should discuss with the undertaker whether burial or cremation is to take place and what his charges will be and what they cover.

The most serious problems arise after the funeral. After the funeral, the full extent of the shock and loss are felt most deeply. It is a time for gritting one's teeth and hanging on by one's fingernails. To cope during this time, try to keep yourself occupied. You probably will want to be alone with your own thoughts, but don't spend all your time alone. Allow other people to help. Don't be ashamed of crying or showing emotion; it's better than keeping your grief bottled up. If you feel that you need tranquilizers or sleeping tablets for a while, ask your doctor. If anything is worrying you about the final illness, do not hesitate to ask the doctor about that as well. Finally, if important decisions about the future have to be made as a result of the death, don't rush into them; let things settle before committing yourself to any far-reaching course of action.

7.

How to Stay Healthy

Although we all must die, death is tragic when it happens as a result of a disease that could have been prevented. Chronic ill health and permanent disability that arise from a preventable disorder are no less tragic. It is important to realize that we now can prevent a great many common conditions and thereby successfully avoid the unnecessarily early disability and death to which they all too frequently lead. To do so, we must understand man's basic needs as well as the ways to control disease and the ways to improve or maintain our fitness and health.

Our Basic Needs

Man cannot, of course, stay alive for long without food, water, oxygen, sleep, and efficiently functioning organs and systems, plus clothing and shelter. He also needs a mind that organizes his activities so he can obtain things he requires for his survival and well-being. Beyond that, he hopes for and aspires to a life that is more than mere subsistence. He seeks happiness. As man's physical necessities become more or less assured, he devotes more time and energy to the pursuit of happiness. Some of the strivings for happiness have been part of man's nature since the time of Adam; others have begun to play a much greater role since the coming of the age of affluence. Certainly nowadays, man's emotional requirements take up much of his time and energy, and emotional disorders or frustrations probably account for more illness than physical disease.

The most basic form of mental, emotional, or psychological activity is instinct. Instincts are inborn tendencies, almost demands, for us and other animals to behave in certain ways when faced with a particular set of circumstances. These instincts are biologically designed to protect and preserve first our own lives and second the lives of the group, be it family, herd, or species, to which we belong. Since many instincts are lifesaving, they are so deeply ingrained that they are almost automatic. We have little control over such instincts and find it difficult to deny or fight them.

The universal instincts, in animals as well as men, concern self-protection and the preservation of life. For instance, obtaining food and drink and reproducing are primary instincts, since without them, we as individuals and mankind as a species would perish. These instincts are overriding forces that sweep aside, when the circumstances demand it, every obstacle in their path regardless of the risk or cost.

Secondary instincts are not as demanding as the primary ones. They are not as vital to man's survival, but for most people they are vital to happiness. The first of these is the instinct for power. This instinct drives people to compete and try to gain positions of superiority over others in terms of achievement, wealth, or position. The second is the herd instinct. The herd instinct leads people to think and act in groups and communities. The third is the spiritual instinct. This instinct urges people to reach for goals that are nonselfish, idealistic, and at least materially unrewarding.

The primary and secondary instincts are the major driving forces in most people's lives. Satisfying them without conflict or restraint gives people a sense of security and emotional contentment. The inability to satisfy these instincts, on the other hand, leads to mental tension and pain. Mental tension and pain, if severe enough, will cause some form of emotional or physical illness. The likelihood of an emotional or physical illness depends on the extent to which an instinct has been frustrated. It also depends on the person's mental "strength" and capacity for adapting to adversity and the availability of an alternative form of satisfaction. People differ enormously in the extent to which they are consciously or unconsciously affected by their instincts. And the relative importance of each instinct varies considerably from person to person.

Many of our emotions are related to particular instincts. Fear, for instance, is associated with concern about self-preservation and security; anger, with the need for confrontation and combat; loneliness, with the desire for the company and protection of the "herd"; appetite and hunger, with the need for regular nourishment; sexual desire, with the need to reproduce future generations. As you can see from these examples, the satisfaction of instincts leads to pleasurable, happy feelings; while their frustration results in pain.

The frustration of instincts and other desires also leads to conflict. Though born of frustration and dissatisfaction, conflict is the mainspring of human endeavor and progress. Conflict occurs whenever what we want to do is not immediately possible. What we want to do may put us on a collision course with another person who is after the same goal. Or it may be incompatible with the interests of the herd or the rules of the community in which we live. Or it may represent a struggle with a limitation that is imposed by our bodies, such as illness or disability, or a battle against an obstacle that has been imposed by the world around us, such as drought or flood. We all are frequently involved in situations that lead to conflict with ourselves or with others. Conflict is an inevitable and inescapable part of human life.

But conflict need not be destructive; it can be constructive and creative.

We may react to conflict in four possible ways. We may be successful and victorious; we may submit; we may try to escape; or we may be trapped in conflict indefinitely. In all these reactions to conflict, there are three classes of response—those that are accepted as normal, those that seem to be excessive or exaggerated, and those that are definitely not normal. The difference between them, however, is one of degree because the response that occurs depends partly on the importance and intensity of the conflict and partly on the person involved. Thus, in relation to submission, it is not abnormal for people to submit to their parents and teachers, to the demands of the herd in matters of law and order, or to the conventions of the community regarding acceptable behavior. It is inappropriately excessive, however, for people to feel inferior, unworthy, or guilty over submission in small matters. And it is abnormal for people to feel persistently depressed, or have prolonged feelings of melancholy or of persecution. With escape as a response to conflict, we regard jokes, hobbies, holidays, and fantasy in plays and films as acceptable responses. But we find heavy drinking, drug taking, and outbursts of temperamental behavior excessive responses, and we consider alcoholism and suicidal attempts as abnormal responses.

Instincts as the fundamental driving forces in men's minds are a basic mental activity and result in "primitive" and uncontrolled behavior. But the mind of man is capable of reason, conscious choice, and restraint. The difference between human and animal minds is man's ability to form and hold ideas and relate them to one another. Thus the distinguishing characteristic of higher forms of human mental activity is the idea or thought or concept. Closely related to the capacity to form ideas is man's ability to learn. Animals learn by imitation and by trial and error. Man can benefit from experience in the same way, but he has a greater capacity for memory, which extends the amount he is able to learn and remember, and has greatly increased powers of reasoning, which give him superior powers of choosing intelligently among several courses of action.

Not all minds work, or react, in the same way, nor do they have the same priorities. The marked differences in the function and "shape" of people's minds make up their personality. Personality distinguishes people from one another in a way that is even more fundamental than the differences in the shapes of their bodies and the way they look. What sort of personality we develop—what we become—depends on the characteristics we inherit from our parents and their ancestors and the events we experience in the course of our lives.

What becomes of us also depends on another element, the final side that completes what I call the "triangle of health." This element includes our personal environment of family, friends, education, leisure, housing, work, and income and the needs that are associated with them. It involves what is now called social health.

Man, as we have seen, is an animal that can lead an independent life. He also is a social creature, however. He needs to live as a self-determining individual and as a member of a herd or community. The need to live in a community is not only instinctive and emotional but physical. Because of the development of specialized jobs in the modern world, we rely upon many other people for the necessities of life. Few people today are able to survive for long outside the herd.

Living as a member of a community or society requires giving and taking. To some extent, people's needs vary according to their temperament and interests. But there are some basic needs that we all share and that we expect the community to provide. If it fails to provide these rights, we feel "deprived," and deprivation or social starvation is the basis of social ill health.

What are these basic social needs? The first is money, or more precisely, the essential goods and services that money can buy—food, clothing, housing, heat, light, etc. Normally we expect to work in exchange for money to buy the goods and services that we require. But we also expect society to provide for our basic needs if, through disability, retirement, or a lack of jobs, we cannot work.

We also have come to expect our needs for safety to be met by society. We expect society to arrange for sewage disposal and refuse collection; fire, police, and national defense; education; and health and social services.

Finally, as members of a supposedly civilized and affluent society, we need, or at least expect, to have a good standard of living, one that exceeds subsistence but one that is average for our society in terms of housing, goods, and amenities.

These needs are primarily of a material nature. We have another need which is much less definite but no less important to our health and happiness: the need to be respected. We need two kinds of respect—self-respect and the respect of others—both of which are related to integrity, achievement, and status.

If any of these needs is not met, we feel that we have been deprived of our "rights" or that life has handicapped us in some way. The feeling of deprivation may lead to ill health, which is thus social in origin. Poverty in childhood, inadequate education, poor housing conditions, and unemployment can easily lead to social ill health.

Man has other social needs that must be met if he is to remain healthy and happy. These needs arise from his relationships with other members of the herd and particularly with those closest to him. From our point of view, each of us stands in the center of circles of relationships with other people. The smallest and closest circle is composed of our immediate family; the next is composed of our extended family, including grandparents, aunts, uncles, and cousins. We have other relationships with our neighbors, friends, colleagues at work, and associates in other activities. The circles get wider and wider as they cover our relationships with people in our town or county, our country, our world. We are members of all these groups, and we are related to all the other members in some degree. In each group, we have rights and responsibilities; in each, we can feel wanted, appreciated, and satisfied, but if we don't we will be unhappy and may, as a consequence, develop ill health.

Our physical, emotional, and social needs do not exist separately or in isolation from one another. Nor do they function separately or independently. They act in relation to each other. So what we do and what we become depends on all three. We easily can see how a physical problem, such as a permanent disability, might affect our emotional health because it bars us from doing many kinds of work and from engaging in some leisure activities. We cannot so easily see how social problems, such as unemployment or a broken home, and emotional problems can bring about bodily illness. In reality, however, our state of mind, which depends on social and emotional satisfaction, has a marked effect on the function of many parts of the body and can elicit physical disease.

Thus good health is a triangle that has as its sides physical, emotional, and social conditions. If any side of the triangle is damaged, the whole is threatened, and the stability of the other two sides is in danger. Damage to any side of the triangle results in illness.

Many episodes of illness involve all sides of the triangle of health; many are brought about by a combination of physical, emotional, and social causes. For instance, during a bout of influenza, we have the physical symptoms of a fever, cough, and body aches. We also feel depressed because of the physical illness and its influence on our social well-being through the loss of wages or the lack of social contact.

For most people, an attack of influenza will be over in a week. For some, it will linger but eventually go away. For a few, it will get worse and develop into bronchitis or pneumonia. What happens is not solely contingent on the virulence of the germs or the intensity of the infection or even on the general physical health or "resistance" of the patient. Regardless of the strength of the infection or the physical condition of the person involved, somebody who is depressed because of a recent divorce, for instance, or somebody who is unhappy at work or who has a housing problem is much more likely to develop complications than the contentedly married person who is doing a job he enjoys and is living where he wants.

How Things Go Wrong

Especially when we are in the prime of life and accustomed to good health, we think of ourselves as being definitely well or definitely ill; fit for work or not fit for work. And we think of illnesses and diseases, particularly if we have a name for them, as precise, clearly identifiable conditions that we certainly have or certainly don't have. We may accept difficulties in arriving at a diagnosis or in putting the right label on an illness in the early stages of a disease when it may not have developed enough to be clearly identified. But once the disease is labeled, we believe it will behave predictably and that its treatment will have a predictable outcome.

Doctors today, however, are taking a different view of illness and the way it behaves. They are beginning to understand that emotional and social factors, as well as the physical condition of the patient, play an important role in the cause, pattern, progress, and outcome of episodes of ill health. They are recognizing that conditions such as depression, delinquency, and "family problems" are also "diseases" that require treatment. The concept that a particular disease is a clearly defined and unchanging entity no longer corresponds to what doctors find in practice. Doctors have seen many diseases substantially change in their characteristics over the years. Thus doctors have the tendency today to consider ill health in individuals and world patterns of disease in terms of "disease situations." They look on disease processes and patterns of behavior as dynamic, not static. Of course, all cases of pneumonia or high blood pressure or cancer of the lung have many common features and must be treated in broadly similar ways. However, doctors are more conscious of and concentrate more on the differences in individual cases, particularly in the causes and patterns of development of disease, because these differences may hold important clues for improvement in management and prevention of illness.

Many other factors must be taken into the consideration of illness. Although we think of ourselves as being generally well or ill, we also are aware of subtle changes in our health, such as being "bursting with health" on one day or being "out of sorts" on another. People move from wellness to illness along a sliding scale that has no precisely identifiable measurements and that is affected by scores of factors. We cannot accurately plot our position on this scale because our position constantly changes. Measurements of average human structure and function have limited relevance to individuals whose bodies and minds work normally within a surprisingly wide range of the average values for the population as a whole. In an individual, there is no sharp dividing line between a healthy and a diseased state; often illness and health cannot be clearly separated. What's more, individuals assess their health subjectively, and determinations of good health vary widely from one individual to another.

Patterns of disease vary in other ways, too. First, the picture will change depending on the stage of development of the condition and the progress that has been made with its treatment. Second, variations arise because of the severity of the attack and the age of the patient; the very young and the very old are particularly vulnerable to serious disease.

Variations related to age are, however, only examples of another factor in the constant battle between man and the hostile elements in his environment. This factor is the strength or the "seeds" of disease, the tenacity of the bacteria, cancer cells, stress, of injury, as opposed to the strength of the "soil," the power the body is able to bring to the challenge. The equation between the "seed" and the "soil" is vitally important to an understanding of the causation and prevention of illness. If the disease is extremely strong or virulent, our defenses probably will not be able to prevent illness, no matter how healthy we are or how strong our "resistance" is. Our defenses will effectively resist a weak or mild form of disease unless we have become debilitated in body or mind. Most of our battles with disease fall in between these two extremes, and the outcome of any illness hinges on the strength and deployment of the opposing forces: the extent to which the disease can jeopardize the function of vital organs and the capacity of the body to call upon powerful defense mechanisms.

The "picture" presented by a disease may be altered by other factors. People used to believe that each disease had a single cause, that each illness was a response to a single stimulus or the result of a single area of malfunction. This belief has been replaced by the understanding that most disease situations, even the most overwhelming and apparently sudden outbreaks, originate from disturbances of equilibrium in several different areas. These disturbances increase, perhaps over a long period of time, and eventually culminate in a breakdown in health. The pattern that breakdown presents is based on which of the patient's physical or mental functions have been disturbed, the depth of the disturbance, and the relation of the disturbance to physical or mental functions.

Since the pattern of a man's life responds to changes in the environment and changes in his aspirations, it is not surprising that the pattern of his disease changes, too. Bacteria and other agents of disease are dominated by the impulse to survive, by the drive to adapt adverse aspects of their environment, and by the forces of evolution. Consequently diseases change. As a result of medical advances, some diseases, such as tuberculosis, smallpox, and typhoid, become much less common or disappear altogether. The advances made in medical science from year to year may make diseases considered incurable today to be completely conquered tomorrow. As a result of changes in man's ways of life, other diseases become more prevalent or virulent. For example, diseases related to stress, such as high blood pressure and coronary heart disease, are more common than before.

Sometimes apparently new diseases, such as Legionnaire's

disease, emerge. Occasionally a disorder, such as a virulent strain of an infectious disease, a food contaminant, or an environmental pollutant, suddenly affects a large number of people in a community. Such an outbreak is called an epidemic; the usually widespread and continual occurrence of sporadic cases of a particular disease is called endemic.

What are the most common killing diseases today? Disorders of the heart and circulation, including high blood pressure and strokes, are by far the worst offenders. Various forms of cancer make up the second largest group. Alcoholism and respiratory diseases, such as pneumonia and bronchitis, are also high on the list. Another increasingly important cause of death, especially among young people, is accidents. Disorders of the circulatory system and respiratory diseases, including colds and influenza, are the common causes of nonfatal illnesses. In recent years, there also have been marked increases in mental and emotional disorders, such as anxiety and depression. Although some of these diseases are outside of our control, most are not. And many of these illnesses can be prevented.

PREVENTING DISEASE

There are two broad categories of preventive medicine: public health or community medicine, which ensures that water is pure, food is safe, and waste and refuse are disposed of; and personal health, which involves the actions taken by individuals. Although the maintenance of high standards of public health is vital to the safety of the community and the health of us all, public health's contribution to saving lives has already been achieved in most developed countries. It is unlikely that new advances in public health will further reduce mortality rates. But the personal health field could have a substantial impact on mortality rates.

"Personal health" today has the greatest potential in the crusade against unnecessary death and disability. Personal health care holds the promise of saving more lives than technological medical advances. What's more, the field of personal health care is not waiting for a crucial new discovery or a major breakthrough in technique. All that is necessary to be effective is already known. That knowledge is waiting for us to take note of it, act on it, and save ourselves and our families a great deal of needless pain and trouble in the years to come.

Many illnesses can be prevented by changing our habits, styles of life, and attitudes. More than ever before, whether we have good or bad health during our lives primarily depends on our own actions.

As with so much in the saga of man's unceasing battle with disease and his determination to stay healthy, it is a matter of "seed" and "soil." We must keep away from unnecessary health hazards so the "seeds" of illness have no chance to be sown, and we must maintain the "soil" of our bodies and minds at the peak of health so we are able to resist disease. Preventive medicine and its handmaiden, health education, involve persuading people to use common sense in the care of their health. Preventive medicine's aim is not to establish long lists of "don'ts," promote health fads, or breed hypochondriacs. Preventive medicine seeks to liberate people from the tyranny of unnecessary and pointless death and disability. One way of sidestepping trouble is, of course, to never take any risks. You can avoid getting run down by a car by never crossing the road. That attitude is not being suggested here. But the program that is presented in the next chapter does not recommend becoming so health-, diet-, or cleanliness-conscious that life is a bore. The program presents a balanced view of ways to avoid some of the health hazards to which we expose ourselves and our families and friends. And it involves two kinds of activity: acting to "stay on top," which means keeping one's body and mind in the best possible shape, and avoiding trouble, which is largely a matter of paying attention to the body's warning system and preventing accidents.

8.

Staying on Top

How to Avoid
the Common Killers

Disease	Cause	How to Avoid or Detect the Disease Early
Heart disease	Stress Obesity Smoking	Reduce stress Lose weight Stop smoking Increase exercise
Strokes or high blood pressure	Stress Obesity	Reduce stress Lose weight Increase exercise Check blood pressure regularly
Alcoholism	Overindulgence	Stop drinking alcoholic beverages or drink in moderation
Respiratory disease, such as chronic bronchitis	Smoking	Stop smoking Increase exercise
Lung cancer	Smoking	Stop smoking
Breast cancer		Examine the breasts regularly
Other cancers		Pay attention to any abnormality
Accidents	Carelessness	Caution

The table on the previous page can tell you what the future may have in store for you more accurately than any fortune-teller or horoscope. What is even more important, it tells you what to do if you want to prevent these common diseases. common diseases.

What stands out with startling clarity is that even these major killers are commonly caused by no more than three factors in the environment, and all three can be avoided. Obesity, smoking, and stress are the major villains. Their control will almost guarantee you an extra ten years of healthy, happy living. Since they are so important, we will look at each in detail.

Obesity

Obviously your weight depends on your height, but it also varies with the size of your "frame." Big-boned, broad-shouldered, wide-hipped people are proportionately heavier, and men weigh more than women of the same height. In spite of that:

- If you find it difficult to squeeze into some of your old clothes, you're fat.
- If your flesh moves like jelly when you jump up and down in front of a mirror, you're fat.
- If you pinch the skin at the back of your upper arm, halfway between shoulder and elbow, and the fold is more than an inch thick, you're very fat.

Now check your actual weight, using the charts on page 141. Find your height, then run your finger across the chart until you come to your weight and frame.

- If you are borderline or heavy, read on and do something about it today.
- If you are borderline, make up your mind to check your weight once a week. Weigh yourself on the same scale at the same time of day and in the same amount of clothing.

Height/Weight Guide for Women

Height*		Small Frame		Medium Frame		Large Frame	
in.	cm.	lb.	kg.	lb.	kg.	lb.	kg.
'0"	— 182.9	138-148	62.6-67.1	144-159	65.3-72.1	153-173	69.4-78.5
'11"	— 180.3	134-144	60.8-65.3	140-155	63.5-70.3	149-168	67.6-76.2
'10"	— 177.8	130-140	59.0-63.5	136-151	61.7-68.5	145-163	65.8-74.0
'9"	— 175.3	126-135	57.2-61.2	132-147	59.9-66.7	141-158	64.0-71.7
'8"	— 172.7	121-131	54.9-59.4	128-143	58.1-64.9	137-154	62.1-69.9
'7"	— 170.2	118-127	53.5-57.6	124-139	56.2-63.1	133-150	60.3-68.1
'6"	— 167.6	114-123	51.7-55.8	120-135	54.4-61.2	129-146	58.5-66.2
'5"	— 165.1	111-119	50.3-54.0	116-130	52.6-59.0	125-142	56.7-64.4
'4"	— 162.6	108-116	49.0-52.6	113-126	51.3-57.2	121-138	54.9-62.6
'3"	— 160.0	105-113	47.6-51.3	110-122	49.9-55.3	118-134	53.5-60.8
'2"	— 157.5	102-110	46.3-49.9	107-119	48.5-54.0	115-131	52.2-59.4
'1"	— 154.9	99-107	44.9-48.5	104-116	47.2-52.6	112-128	50.8-58.1
'0"	— 152.4	96-104	45.3-47.2	101-113	45.8-51.3	109-125	49.4-56.7
'11"	— 149.8	94-101	42.6-45.8	98-110	44.4-49.9	106-122	48.1-55.3
'10"	— 147.3	92-98	41.7-44.4	96-107	43.5-48.5	104-119	47.2-54.0

ote: For women between 18 and 25, subtract 1 pound for each year under 25.
Vith shoes with 2-inch heels.

h charts adapted from desirable weight table of the Metropolitan Life Insurance Company.

Height/Weight Guide for Men

Height*		Small Frame		Medium Frame		Large Frame	
1.	cm.	lb.	kg.	lb.	kg.	lb.	kg.
4"	— 193.0	164-175	74.4-79.4	172-190	78.0-86.2	182-204	82.6-92.6
3"	— 190.5	160-171	72.6-77.6	167-185	75.3-83.9	178-199	80.8-90.3
2"	— 188.0	156-167	70.8-75.8	162-180	73.5-81.7	173-194	78.5-88.0
1"	— 185.4	152-162	69.0-73.5	158-175	71.7-79.4	168-189	76.2-85.8
0"	— 182.9	148-158	67.1-71.7	154-170	69.9-77.1	164-184	74.4-83.5
11"	— 180.3	144-154	65.3-69.9	150-165	68.1-74.9	159-179	72.1-81.2
10"	— 177.8	140-150	63.5-68.1	146-160	66.2-72.6	155-174	70.3-78.9
9"	— 175.3	136-145	61.7-65.8	142-156	64.4-70.3	151-170	68.5-77.1
8"	— 172.7	132-141	59.9-64.0	138-152	62.6-69.0	147-166	66.7-75.3
7"	— 170.2	128-137	58.1-62.1	134-147	60.8-66.7	142-161	64.4-73.0
6"	— 167.6	124-133	56.2-60.3	130-143	59.0-64.9	138-156	62.6-70.8
5"	— 165.1	121-129	54.9-58.5	127-139	57.6-63.1	135-152	61.2-69.0
4"	— 162.6	118-126	53.5-57.2	124-136	56.2-61.7	132-148	59.9-67.1
3"	— 160.0	115-123	52.2-55.8	121-133	54.9-60.3	129-144	58.5-65.3
2"	— 157.5	112-120	50.8-54.4	118-129	53.5-58.5	126-141	57.2-64.0

th shoes with 1-inch heels.   heim, L   ⁴ N.Y. ¹

Why all the fuss about being overweight? Obesity is one of the most common killers today. It reduces life expectancy by as much as 40 percent. It can cause arteriosclerosis, heart disease, coronary artery disease, gall-bladder disease, high blood pressure, and strokes from the added strain put on the circulation; and it can bring on arthritis and varicose veins from the added load on the legs. Many of these conditions, even when they are not fatal, cause severe and permanent disability. Obese people also are much more likely to have accidents because they are less nimble, and they are at greater risk of complications during pregnancy or following an operation.

How do people become overweight? Diseases that lead to obesity are rare. Actually, in ninety-nine out of one hundred cases, people became overweight by eating more food—especially more carbohydrates and fats—than their bodies could use. The equation is a simple one. If the food eaten exceeds the food used, the balance will be stored as fat. Lack of exercise plays a part because exercise can alter the equation by increasing the amount of food that is used up.

Those who obviously overeat are not the only ones who become fat. Those who eat slightly more than is needed eventually will have a weight problem. People are not equally affected, however. Some seem to be able to eat what they like without putting on weight; others have difficulty keeping their weight under control. These traits appear to be hereditary. The tendency to become overweight increases with age; the critical period is the forties. But this relationship with age may reflect people's tendency to eat more and exercise less as they grow older.

Why do people overeat? In most cases, people overeat because eating tasty foods, especially those that are sweet, is pleasurable. Generally the tastiest foods and drinks are the most dangerous for the overweight. Cravings for such foods are easy to develop, and eating them can become a habit or even an addiction, particularly for people whose lives are unsatisfying in other ways or for those who are lonely, unhappy, or depressed. Such people tend to eat because they can rely on the pleasure of eating; they know eating will not let them down.

Eating large meals is a regular part of many people's social and working lives, and it is not surprising that they become overweight. Some people get caught in a vicious circle of hopelessness about their weight. They alternate crash diets with binges and trade feelings of elation for guilt. They usually end up feeling angry and resentful because they seem to be trapped with a steadily deteriorating weight problem.

Are you overweight? Check your weight and height on the chart on page 141. (Note that there is no allowance for age if you are over 25.) How do you measure up against the chart? If you are ten percent overweight according to the chart, you should beware. If you are twenty percent overweight, you are in danger and probably would not receive life insurance at normal rates. If you are thirty percent or more overweight, you are almost certain to die well before your time or to develop a permanently disabling disease unless you do something *now*.

How to lose weight. For most people losing weight is difficult and, since it involves giving up foods and drinks that they like very much, it also is unpleasant. There are no easy ways and no short cuts to losing weight. Determination and willpower are important. So are a clear idea of why losing weight is necessary and an understanding of the equation that governs weight gain. But success is rewarded by improved health and appearance and by a feeling of extreme satisfaction.

No long-term weight loss can be achieved without a change, often a drastic one, in eating habits. A vague intention to diet by cutting down on this or that is never enough. On the other hand, it is not necessary to be chained to a calorie chart and add to the boredom of figuring out the calories in every meal the pain of going without some favorite foods. It is wise, however, to have a chart to check on the calories of broad food categories and particular items. The chart on pages 144–48 shows the calorie value of moderate portions of some common foods.

Calorie Chart

Meat	Oz.	Cal.
Bacon, lean (3 slices)	2	250
Beef, Burgers (2 patties)	3	120
Sirloin, lean, roast	3	200
Steak, stewed	3	190
Brains, calf, boiled	3	78
Chicken, boiled (3 slices)	3	130
Chicken, roast (3 slices)	3	126
Corned beef (2 slices)	1½	91
Ham, lean, boiled (1 slice)	1½	93
Heart, sheep, roast	3	204
Kidney, stewed	3	78
Lamb chops, broiled (1 medium)	4	310
Lamb, roast (3 slices)	3	246
Pork chops (1 medium)	4	375
Rabbit, stewed	3	153
Sausages (2 large)	4	400
Turkey, roast (2 slices)	3	168
Veal cutlet, roast	3	189

Fish		
Cod, broiled	3	135
Cod, fried	3	150
Cod, steamed	4	92
Crab, boiled	3	108
Haddock, fried	3	150
Haddock, steamed	3	84
Halibut	3	111
Herrings, fried (1 small)	3	201
Lobster, boiled (1 medium)	3	102
Mackerel, fried	3	159
Mussels, boiled	3	75
Oysters	3	42

Fish Cont.	Oz.	Cal.
Prawns	3	90
Rock salmon, fried	3	200
Salmon, canned	3	132
Sardines, canned (4 large)	3	186
Shrimps	3	96
Sole, fried (1 medium fillet)	3	200
Sole, steamed (1 medium fillet)	3	72
Trout, steamed	3	106
Turbot, steamed	3	84
Whiting, steamed	3	78

Fruit		
Apple (1 medium)	4	52
Apricots (2 small)	4	32
Apricots, canned (6 halves and syrup)	4	120
Avocado (1 fruit)	6	150
Banana (1 medium)	6	132
Cherries (½ cup)	4	55
Grapefruit (½ fruit)	3	18
Grapes (1 cup)	2	34
Melon (2″ wedge)	3	18
Orange (1 medium)	4	40
Peach (1 medium)	4	45
Peaches, canned (3 halves and syrup)	4	100
Pear (1 medium)	5	55
Pears, canned (2 halves and syrup)	4	80
Pineapple (1 medium slice)	2	26
Pineapple, canned (2 slices and juice)	4	88
Plum (1 large)	2	18
Raspberries (1 cup)	4	28
Rhubarb (1 cup)	4	8
Strawberries (1 cup)	4	30
Tangerine (1 medium)	1½	15

Nuts		
Almonds (12 nuts)	1	165

Nuts Cont.	Oz.	Cal.
Brazil nuts (6 nuts)	1	175
Coconut, dessicated (3 tsp.)	1	173
Peanuts	1	171
Walnuts (8 nuts)	2	312

Vegetables		
Artichoke, boiled (1 small)	4	15
Asparagus	4	20
Beans, baked, canned (½ cup)	4	80
Beans, butter, boiled	4	104
Beans, butter, raw	2	152
Beans, French, boiled (4 tbsp.)	4	8
Beans, string, boiled (4 tbsp.)	4	250
Beets, raw	4	52
Beets, boiled (6 slices)	4	48
Broccoli (boiled)	4	16
Brussels sprouts, boiled (5 large)	4	20
Cabbage, boiled (4 tbsp.)	4	20
Carrots, raw or boiled (4 tbsp.)	4	20
Cauliflower, boiled (4 tbsp.)	4	15
Celery, boiled (3 medium sticks)	4	4
Celery, raw (3 medium sticks)	4	12
Cucumber, raw (6 large slices)	2	4
Leeks, boiled (1 stick)	4	28
Lentils, boiled (1 cup)	4	108
Lettuce (6 large leaves)	4	12
Mushrooms, fried	2	124
Mushrooms, raw	4	8
Onions, fried (½ vegetable)	2	200
Onions, raw (1 medium)	4	28
Peas, canned (4 tbspl)	4	88
Peas, fresh, boiled (4 tbsp.)	4	52
Potato chips (10 large)	4	270
Potatoes, baked (2 medium)	4	130
Potatoes, boiled (2 medium)	4	92
Potatoes, mashed (3 medium)	4	116

Vegetables Cont.	Oz.	Cal.
Radishes, raw (8 small)	2	8
Spinach, boiled (4 tbsp.)	4	28
Tomatoes, raw (2 medium)	4	16
Watercress	2	8

Dairy Products		
Butter (2 pats)	1	207
Cheese, Cheddar (1″ cube)	1	120
Cheese, cottage (1 tsp.)	1	32
Cheese, cream	1	232
Cream (2 tsp.)	2	262
Egg, boiled (1 large)	2	84
Egg, fried (1 large)	2½	170
Egg, poached (1 large)	2	90
Lard (2 tsp.)	1	254
Margarine (2 tsp.)	1	208
Milk (½ pint)	10	190
Milk, condensed	1½	140
Oil (1½ tsp.)	1	255
Yogurt, low fat (1 carton)	4	60

Grain Foods		
Barley, boiled	2	68
Bread, brown (1 slice, ½″ thick)	1	65
Bread, white, toasted (1 slice, ¾″ thick)	1	85
Bread, whole wheat (1 slice, ½″ thick)	1	68
Cake, sponge (1 slice)	2	164
Corn flakes (1 cup)	1	100
Doughnut	1	202
Jelly roll	2	230
Macaroni (½ cup)	4	102
Oatmeal (2 tsp.)	2	226
Pancakes (1 medium)	2	170
Pastry, flaky	2	334
Pie, Fruit (1 slice)	3	160
Pie, Mince (1 slice)	2	222

Grain Foods Cont.	Oz.	Cal.
Puffed wheat	1	102
Rice (½ cup)	4	400
Shredded wheat	1	103
Spaghetti (½ cup)	4	410

Drinks

	Oz.	Cal.
Beer (1 pint)		240
Champagne (1 glass)		125
Chocolate milk (1 cup)		180
Cider (½ pint)		120
Cocoa (2 tsp. in water)	1	128
Coffee, instant (1 tsp. in water)	¼	11
Coffee (1 tsp. in water)	½	20
Lemon juice (1 glass)	4	10
Lemonade (1 glass)		48
Mineral water (1 glass)		48
Alcohol (large-measure shot)		126
Tea, milk, no sugar (1 cup)		20
Tea, no milk or sugar (1 cup)		0
Wine, dry (1 glass)		100
Wine, sweet (1 glass)		120

Miscellaneous

	Oz.	Cal.
Chocolate bar, milk or plain (1 bar)	4	620
Cornstarch (1 tsp.)	1	100
Curry powder (1 tsp.)	½	33
Flour (1½ tsp.)	1	98
Ground ginger (1 tsp.)	½	28
Honey (1 tsp.)	2	164
Ice cream (1 scoop)	2	110
Jam or marmalade (1 tsp.)	2	148
Soup, cream (1 cups)		180
Sugar (4 tsp.)	1	112
Syrup (1 tsp)	2	168
Tomato sauce (½ cup)	4	101

Many people lose weight quite satisfactorily by consuming 1,000 calories a day, but you should not consume fewer than 800 calories a day unless your doctor advises it. Do not jump from overeating to a strict 800-calorie-a-day diet overnight. Start at 1,200 calories and work down over the next ten days. And do check with your doctor to see if there is any reason why you should not try to lose weight.

The calorie limit that you adopt should be related to the work you do and to the degree to which you are overweight. If you are very overweight and have an office job, you may work down to a diet of 800 calories a day. If you have an office job and are only moderately overweight, a 900-calorie-a-day diet will do. A 900-calorie-a-day diet also will work for somebody who does heavy work and is extremely overweight.

The following diet is easy to follow and suitable for anyone. It contains all essential nutrients and offers a wide choice of foods; yet it is effective in losing weight.

On this diet, you may eat as much as you like of:

- Lean meat, rabbit, bacon, ham, and poultry
- Fish
- Eggs
- Cottage cheese
- Salads
- Vegetables, except potatoes
- Fruit of all kinds except bananas, grapes, dried or canned fruit, and fruit dishes prepared with sugar
- Tea, coffee, water, and bouillon

You may consume limited amounts of:

- Milk (up to a half-pint a day)
- Butter, margarine, or cream (one tablespoon a day)
- Starch-reduced bread (up to six rolls or three ounces of bread a day)
- Cereals (one small helping of breakfast cereal, rice, macaroni, or spaghetti *instead of* one-third of the ration of bread)

● Cheeses other than cottage cheese (one one-inch cube a day)

You may eat *nothing else.* Beware of nibbling between meals, sugar in disguise, cocktail and television snacks, nuts, thick soups and sauces, sausages, ice cream, and other desserts.

What you should aim for is a gradual, steady, and sustained weight loss. How long you take to get down to the weight you want may vary, but weight loss usually takes from one to three months. The rate at which people lose weight differs; so don't despair if you are progressing more slowly than some of your friends. But don't become overly scale-conscious. Variations of a few pounds either way occur naturally from day to day, and they usually are of no significance. A weekly weigh-in is sufficient, but do try to use the same scale at the same time of day and wear similar clothes. Don't become a calorie bore. If you go out to a special dinner and exceed your calorie limit, cut back that amount over the next three days. And don't feel you need to be hungry. Make sure that you always have something filling on hand. A few carrots or apples are very effective standbys for many dieters. Once you have reached your ideal weight, you must stay there. It is all too easy to let your weight slide upward again, and it is worth taking the trouble to keep an eye on what you eat.

What about exercise? Although increased exercise is a great help to dieting and your overall health, you cannot slim sufficiently by exercising alone. A half-hour of swimming or tennis or three-quarters of an hour of cycling or walking three miles a day will burn up three pounds a month. But that amount of exercise accomplishes the same as avoiding thirteen lumps of sugar or four slices of bread.

Losing weight is seldom easy. Here are a few things that can help.

Involve your family and friends so they give you meals that you can finish. Get into the habit of making your food go as far as possible by cutting it into small pieces and eating it slowly. And remember there is absolutely no limit on the amount of water that you can drink.

Devise monetary rewards appropriate for your level of achievement. Since you probably will spend less on meals than you used to, you can use this money to buy a luxury. Rewards make dieting more fun and make up for some of the eating pleasures you must do without.

Some people find it easier to lose weight in the company of others who have the same problem. If you do, you may try to join such groups as Weight Watchers International, Inc. Some people, no matter how conscientiously they stick to the rules, genuinely find it difficult or impossible to lose weight. If you are one of these, get the help of your doctor. There are several ways in which he may be able to assist you, including special hospital treatments for exceptional cases.

What about drugs? Unfortunately there is no drug that will burn up excess fat and therefore no drug that substitutes for dieting. Most so-called slimming drugs act by diminishing the appetite (anorectics). If hunger is a major problem, you may try an anorectic during the first week or two of dieting before the body's appetite-regulating center has become adjusted to decreased amounts of food. You also should not take appetite suppressants for more than a short time. You may come to rely on them instead of dieting.

Drugs that increase the amount of fluid lost from the body (diuretics) are sometimes used to assist slimmers. These drugs may spur a substantial and encouraging initial loss. However, unless fluid retention is associated with heart or kidney disease, it is not a factor in most cases of obesity. Consequently diuretics have no place in the treatment of obesity. Thyroid preparations have been used to promote weight loss in some people. To be effective, however, they must be given in large doses. Large doses of these drugs speed up the body's machinery, which may be undesirable and cause toxicity. Daily injections of human chorionic gonadotrophin have been used by some doctors. These hormone injections are very expensive and are given to people who are following diets of as little as 500 calories. These extremely low-calorie diets probably are more responsible for the weight loss than the hormone is.

Several other so-called aids to slimming are of little or no value and actually may be harmful. They include Turkish baths and saunas and vibrating exercise machines and "spot reducers."

Are You Eating the Right Food?

Eating sensibly involves more than having neither too much nor too little. You also must be sure that you are getting proper nourishment. The average person eats about a half-ton of food a year. Although the body efficiently extracts what it needs from this massive mixture, it can cope only up to a point. If you go on eating too much of some things and not enough of others, you eventually will get out of condition, and your health and well-being may suffer.

After all, you are what you eat. So think before you eat. The food may look good and may taste good. But how much good is the food doing for you?

Your food should balance your body's need for:

Nutrients (proteins, fats, carbohydrates, vitamins, minerals, and water)—the raw materials needed to build and repair the body-machine.

Energy (calories)—to power the body-machine and the thousands of mechanisms and actions that keep you alive and active.

Dietary fiber (a complex mixture of natural plant substances)—the value of which we are just beginning to understand.

Most people in this country eat more than enough nutrients. Undernutrition is virtually a thing of the past. If you're eating a varied diet, it is just about impossible for you to get too little protein, vitamins, or minerals.

Take protein, for instance. On the average, we eat about twice as much protein as we need. Ignore the television ads for products that have added protein to make you strong and healthy. Extra protein probably won't make any difference.

Vitamin pills probably won't make any difference either. A

varied diet with plenty of fresh fruit, vegetables, and cereals along with some fish, eggs, meat, and dairy products will contain more than enough of all the vitamins. Unless you have a special medical reason, vitamin pills are a waste of time and money.

As for minerals, there is no shortage in the average diet. True, pregnant women and those who have heavy periods may need extra iron (liver, kidneys, and green leafy vegetables are good food sources). But most people eat all the minerals essential for good health.

And chances are you are eating too much of the other nutrients—fats and carbohydrates. Finicky eaters and crash dieters could be ignoring some important nutrient. And nutrient intake may not be sufficient during special times, such as pregnancy, when nutritional requirements change. On the whole, however, lack of nutrients isn't a problem these days. Nor is calorie intake. Except for the slimmers who deliberately cut down on them, most people eat more than enough calories. But because of the abundance of meat, dairy products, and refined foods, many of us may not be getting enough dietary fiber.

Throughout man's evolution, his daily diet came mainly from plants, from unrefined cereals, vegetables, fruits, and nuts; meat was just an occasional delicacy. So over hundreds of thousands of years, our ancestors adapted to food containing a high proportion of dietary fiber. In comparison with our ancestors' diet, the modern Western diet contains relatively little dietary fiber. Most of our diet consists of meat, eggs, and dairy products, which contain no fiber, and we eat few cereal foods, which are a good source of fiber.

Lack of fiber seems to be connected with disorders of the bowels, including hemorrhoids, diverticulitis (a serious inflammation), and constipation, and it may play a role in diabetes, heart disease, and even some types of cancer. In addition, eating more fiber actually may help you to stay slim. A meal containing a high proportion of fiber can be satisfying without filling you up with concentrated calories.

Here are some ways of getting more fiber in your diet:

- Eat more bread, especially whole wheat bread. Whole wheat bread is an underrated food. It is a good, cheap source of fiber and nutrients but has few concentrated calories.
- Eat more potatoes. Potatoes are another underrated food. Potatoes are excellent fillers and need not be fattening if you don't load them with butter or fry them in fat.
- Have a high-fiber cereal for breakfast. The more wheat bran a cereal contains, the higher the fiber content.
- Plan more meals around beans, peas, and lentils. Use meat more sparingly.
- Eat more vegetables, particularly green, leafy ones which are high in fiber. But don't overcook them. Cook them just until they soften slightly.
- Eat plenty of fresh fruits and salads. Even soft fruits such as melon or oranges have fiber. Because fruits and vegetables contain a lot of water, they are low in calories and help you stay slim.
- Make room for all this good food by cutting down on sugary and fatty foods, especially between meals.

SMOKING

There are at least five known cancer-producing substances as well as many other irritating chemicals in cigarette smoke. The chance of developing cancer of the mouth or throat is ten times greater for smokers. The chance of developing cancer of the lung is twenty-five times greater for smokers. Even today, only a few people with lung cancer can be treated effectively by surgery or radiation therapy. In most cases, treatment makes little difference.

Smokers are five or six times more likely to develop chronic bronchitis. Chronic bronchitis is incurable. It leads to increasing shortness of breath and restricted activity. Many patients are so short of breath, they must be confined to their homes or even to their beds.

Smoking also causes heart disease and peptic ulcers. In fact, smokers have double the normal chance of dying from heart disease. Eighty-five out of one hundred nonsmokers live to be 65 or more, but only sixty out of one hundred smokers live to this age. One in four of the people who started smoking before age twenty will die from it. Smoking shortens your life by five and one-half hours every day. It shortens your life by five and one-half minutes each time you smoke a cigarette.

How to Stop Smoking

There are no miracle cures, no magic methods, no short cuts, no foolproof formulas, no alternative to sheer dogged determination. Nevertheless, the battle *can* be won. Several million win it each year, and *you* can, too. As in any battle, success depends on courage, determination, and skillful planning.

Courage comes first. Giving up something that you enjoy and have come to rely on is bound to hurt. The temptation to have just one cigarette, especially if you are under stress, is difficult to resist. But remember, the world is full of people who have given up smoking time and again. It takes courage not to become one of them.

Determination comes second. You must make up your mind before you start that without any "ifs" or "buts" or "maybes" you are going to kick the habit once and for all. A half-hearted attempt or a strategy based on gradually cutting down is almost certain to fail.

To have the best chance of success, you also need planning. Just getting up one morning and saying, "This is the day I give up smoking," may work for some people. But for most, it's a perfect recipe for at most a nine-day nonsmoking campaign. The battle will be tough; so prepare for it. Start at the beginning. Find out why you are giving up smoking. List the reasons you believe smoking is harmful and distasteful as well as any other reasons you have for wanting to stop. Keep the list with you so you can refer to it and strengthen your resolve whenever you are tempted to smoke.

Learn your present smoking pattern. Keep a daily smoking diary for a full week. In the diary, report when and what you were doing when you started a cigarette. Make sure you enter each cigarette. You can easily cheat without meaning to. When you have completed the diary, study it to discover your pattern of smoking: the times of the day and the situations you commonly associate with having a cigarette. These times and situations are going to require special concentration and effort when you give up smoking.

Name your personal F-Day, the day on which you will win freedom from this dangerous and distasteful habit. Plan to stop smoking on a day that probably will be free of stress and worry. All through your campaign, do everything possible to give yourself the best chance of winning. So for the time being, avoid friends who smoke, go to places where you would not be expected to smoke, and use nonsmoking areas of trains, restaurants, etc.

The evening before your F-Day, make sure you have no cigarettes in the house, your clothes, or your car. Remind yourself, from your list of reasons, why you have decided to give up smoking. Think about the day ahead: where you will be and what you will be doing. From your smoking diary, identify the times you will be tempted to have a cigarette. Try to work out in advance how you will resist that temptation.

Before you go to work on F-Day, go through your list of reasons for giving up smoking. Remind yourself that this is possibly the most important battle of your life and that you will win it.

In spite of all your planning, problems will arise. Here's how to deal with the common ones.

If you miss feeling a cigarette in your mouth, have something on hand to suck, nibble, or chew—gum, a carrot, or an apple. If your usual routine is disagreeably disturbed by not smoking (you miss a cigarette with the morning coffee or after a meal), replace smoking with something else or break your routine. Have tea instead of coffee in the morning or go for a stroll after dinner.

If you miss having a cigarette when you feel tense or are worried, try chewing or nibbling on something or try relaxation exercises. Take long, slow, deep breaths and hold them for a count of ten before exhaling. Or let all parts of your body relax while you think about and feel the tension draining out of you.

Although successfully getting through the F-Day is encouraging, the battle is far from over. The days ahead often are tougher to get through than the first one. For most people, the real difficulties, the most insistent temptation to "have just one," the most testing and agonizing moments come at the end of the first week or beginning of the second. At such times, you must recite your reasons for giving up again and again, grit your teeth, and refuse to give in. This period can be real hell, but every cigarette that you refuse is a triumph, and you come closer to the day when refusing a cigarette will no longer be a struggle. That day may come in three to four weeks or longer, especially if there have been lapses along the way. The secret is to take every day, every hour, and possibly every minute as it comes. Don't worry or even think about how you're going to live without a cigarette for the rest of your life or even the rest of the day. Just concentrate on doing without one for the next minute.

Rewards. The best rewards are, of course, cumulative, and they are gained over a period of months and years. Over time, your morning cough will disappear, and you will have fewer colds and chest infections. In the long run, your probable life span will increase. But some rewards begin the moment you stop smoking. For instance, you'll look better and have better senses of smell and taste; your nicotine stains will begin to fade; you will become out of breath less easily; and your stamina will start to improve. If you are pregnant, your baby will immediately have a much better chance of first-class physical and mental health.

You also will start to become richer. Each time you resist the temptation to have a cigarette, put the money you would have paid for it in a special pocket or part of your purse. Or wait until the end of the day, then figure out how much you used to spend on cigarettes and put the money away or at least keep an account of it. This money should be used to buy yourself something you would not otherwise have had; so in addition to your improved health, you will have a tangible reward for not smoking.

Stress—What It Can Do to You and How to Stop It

Mental disorders may lead to madness or insanity and the need for permanent care in a hospital. But most of them are less serious; these illnesses, which are categorized as nervous breakdowns, do not last long and can be treated outside the hospital.

There are many different types of mental disorders, and their causes vary. Some are due to birth defects or to injuries to the brain; some are due to disturbances of the brain's chemical processes; and some are due to as yet unknown causes. Others are the result of excessive emotional stress.

Conflict and stress between ourselves and the world around us are inescapable. Stress serves a useful purpose when it stimulates effort, inventiveness, and the urge to meet high standards. But when there is more stress than we can cope with, it may cause an illness which has mental or physical manifestations. Whether or not we have a breakdown, and how a breakdown affects us, depends on many factors. The most important involves the intensity of the stress to which we are subjected and our capacity to contain and adapt to it. The pressures that result from excessive stress probably are greater in our generation than in previous ones. But our ability to deal with stress hinges on the characteristics we inherited at birth, the experiences we had during our formative years, and the successes and failures we felt in dealing with our environment.

The ability to cope with stress is based on a person's constitutional or natural resources, character, training, and experience. Coping with stress involves certain subconscious defense mechanisms. We may discount or refuse to recognize reality or deny the existence of such unpleasant facts as the breakup of a relationship. We may fail at work or at achieving personal standards and become hostile toward others for our own failings. We may rationalize failure to achieve an objective by trying to convince ourselves that we didn't really want it anyway. We may compensate for our failure in one area by making exceptional achievements in another. We may displace our distress by displaying friendliness and charm when we feel hostility and anxiety.

As with all other health versus illness situations, many elements interact, and the interaction creates a constantly changing picture which may not hold still long enough for us to grasp. Not surprisingly, therefore, most of us find ourselves, our state of mind at any particular time, and our motives confusing. Fortunately the main features of a mental illness usually are clear and last long enough for diagnosis and treatment to be made.

Intense stress is often preceded by excessive anxiety, fear, distress, guilt, or shame. In addition, prolonged, repeated, or severe stress may precipitate disturbances in bodily function, which are called psychosomatic illnesses and include "tension headache," dyspepsia, skin disorders, vaginal discharge, and menstrual problems. Stresses that are fundamentally emotional or social may be self-perpetuating because they alter a person's scale of values and the way he looks at things. Even though reactions to physical diseases differ, most people can agree that a rash is a rash and that raised temperature constitutes a fever. But a depressed person is likely to see himself and the world around him differently than other people do, and his reactions may be disturbed as much by this disorientation as by his depression.

It is important to recognize when things are going wrong and help is needed, since the sufferers of some types of mental illness may not be able to make the determination themselves. The distinction between mental health and mental disorder, sanity and madness, is seldom distinct or easy, but there are some more or less general features of mental health. The first is self-awareness or insight. A mentally well person's assessment of himself, his strengths and weaknesses, and achievements and failures corresponds with facts and with the observations of those around him. He does not substantially under- or overrate himself, and his behavior responds to reality, not to a world of fantasy or delusion. His view of people and events also is "real"; he does not perpetually misperceive situations or motives or appear blind to unpleasant facts.

A mentally well person for the most part can manage his life as an independent person. He is not excessively dominated by or dependent on others. He is able to marshal his mental and physical powers to concentrate or focus on particular tasks. And he is well adjusted. He has control over himself at most times; he makes sensible choices in his life; he accepts the things he cannot change and pursues the possible rather than the impossible; he gains satisfaction from his achievements and is content.

This description may seem to paint a picture of perfection that none of us can match and consequently means all of us are somewhat mad. Certainly we all have the seeds of a nervous breakdown or a mental disorder in us. We would be very dull, and the world's intellectual and cultural progress would stand still, if it were not so. However, the final feature of mental health is the person's successful integration of the different and often dissonant elements in his character so he effectively functions as a balanced, consistent whole.

Substantial departures from these criteria of mental health indicate an emotional problem. Other common pointers often are involuntary cries for help, and they should be regarded as such. The danger signs are:

- Neglect of self-care and personal appearance
- Lack of personal or social relationships, undue isolation, or quarrelsomeness
- Carelessness in relationships as a friend, parent, or lover or in the quality of work

- Absence or deviation of sexual interests
- Disinterest in or inability to work or an overall lack of enthusiasm, drive, or progress
- Persistent feelings of gloominess, melancholy, or depression or an overall lack of hope
- Excessive dependence on or exploitation by others, an "inferiority complex," or undue pliability
- Dependence on or addiction to drugs, alcohol, or tobacco
- Excessive anxiety, irritability, or sleeplessness
- Behavioral abnormalities, including cheating and deceitfulness

Just as pain warns us of physical injury, so unhappiness or mental pain signals injury to our emotional stability. We can feel just as ill when we have an emotional problem as we do when we have a physical problem. Consultation and examination by a doctor usually are necessary to determine if our feelings of ill health are physical or emotional in origin because the reactions of our bodies and minds are much closer than we think. What happens to our bodies clearly has an effect on how we feel; but how we feel often affects the way our bodies function. Fainting is a good example. We may faint because we are physically ill, because we have had a sudden shock, or because we are mentally exhausted or unhappy. Continuing or repeated stress affects the mind and the body as well. Two of the most common and most serious physical results of constant stress are high blood pressure (hypertension) and heart attacks (coronary thrombosis). Other physical results are skin infections and digestive disorders.

From the standpoint of prevention, it is important to understand how a nervous breakdown arises.

What sort of people we are, in both body and mind, depends on what has happened to us. Anxiety is a normal reaction to threatening situations, but if we experienced excessive anxiety and insecurity in early childhood, we may be overanxious in later life. All babies naturally become frustrated, angry, and anxious at times; but the child who is persistently neglected, unloved, and lonely will likely grow into a nervous, anxious, aggressive, and disturbed adolescent. Growing up inevitably brings problems, especially in dealing with parents and other sources of authority, levels of achievement at school and at play, and the upheaval of puberty. How these problems are handled, rather than the problems themselves, is important to future mental health.

Worries and anxieties over work and career, social and sexual relationships, illnesses and bereavements occur from time to time throughout our adult lives. The demands of "civilized" behavior also give rise to tension because they force us to do many things we do not want to do and to forego many things we want. Anxieties and tensions may become so great that work is no longer possible, and the ordered pattern of life disintegrates. Unless help is forthcoming, the strain tends to get worse and may reach the breaking point.

What happens during a nervous breakdown varies considerably. Usually, however, the "coping" mechanisms begin to fail or become overwhelmed by severe, persistent, or repeated stress. When coping mechanisms fail, one or more "danger signs" appear (see pages 160–61). Consultation and counseling at this stage may relieve the problem and prevent it from developing further. If people are able to talk about their problems with someone they respect—a lover, parent, teacher, friend, or doctor—or to share the responsibility for their decisions with others, stress often is greatly reduced. But many people do not seek counseling because they are unaware of what is happening to them, do not appreciate its significance, underestimate their need for help, or refuse to seek assistance for fear of being labeled a "mental case." For these people, the problem intensifies. These people begin to feel surrounded by inescapable, insoluble, and unremitting fears. They despair and lose their sense of purpose and their hope for the future. They are sleepless, unable to communicate with others, withdrawn, isolated, and in limbo. They may mark their actual breaking point by staying in bed or refusing to work or leave the house; by committing an act of aggression; by engaging in an outburst; by attempting suicide; or by acting abnormally in other ways.

The mental disorder to which the breakdown gives rise varies, but it usually is related to the patient's personality. In contrast to the more serious mental disorders, which are called psychoses, the patient who has had a breakdown knows that his reactions and behavior are abnormal but can do nothing about them. He feels as though his actions were out of his control. This type of mental or emotional upset is called a neurosis. It is important to distinguish between the medical meaning of "neurotic," which refers to a particular group of mental illnesses, and the general use of the word as referring to people who are nervous or subject to "imaginary" illnesses.

The first, and probably the most common, type of neurosis is an *anxiety neurosis* or a state of anxiety during which the patient constantly feels apprehensive, fearful, and in dread of impending disaster but is unable to say what alarms him. In particularly severe or sudden forms, these feelings reach a panic state. In panic states, physical "fight or flight" reactions, such as increased and sometimes audible beating of the heart (palpitations), sweating, rapid breathing, trembling, flushing, and overactivity of bladder and bowels, add to the patient's distress. Anxieties also may interfere with the patient's memory so he cannot recall people's names or remember well-known facts.

In phobias or *phobic neurosis,* the patient's fear, though no less irrational and misplaced, relates to something specific, such as fear of public places (agoraphobia) or fear of confined areas (claustrophobia). There are over 130 recognized phobias concerning such subjects as heights, traffic, dogs, cats, birds, spiders, bees, moths, darkness, thunderstorms, matches, knives, and various foods. There also are social phobias, which include fears about eating, drinking, speaking, blushing, or vomiting in the presence of others, and illness phobias, which cover fears of brain tumors, cancer, venereal disease, impotence, and imminent death. The sight of, or likelihood of contact with, the subject of a phobia immediately throws the patient into acute anxiety or panic and sometimes makes him feel unreal and outside himself. The patient, therefore, will go to almost unbelievable lengths to avoid it. Attempts at reasoning with a person who has a phobia actually may increase his distress; he knows that his fear is unreasonable and does not need someone to point that out. Treatment can be extremely difficult, but desensitization has been successful in many cases. In desensitization, the patient, while relaxed, is exposed to what he fears in "doses" that gradually increase from minimal to intense. This therapy has been particularly successful when combined with psychotherapy related to the cause of the phobia.

Hysteria (a hysterical state or *hysterical neurosis*) is quite different from "having an attack of hysterics." An attack of hysterics is a sudden, uncontrolled outburst of pent-up feelings. Hysteria, on the other hand, involves the diversion or conversion of mental conflict and tension into a physical disability, such as a headache or fainting spell, blindness, deafness, or paralysis. After onset of the physical disability, the mental tension dissolves; indeed there often is an incongruous indifference to the disability. The element of "gain" may be specific in that the disability effectively resolves a conflict, at least temporarily—for instance, when a child with a problem at school on Thursdays regularly develops stomach pains on Wednesday nights. A different type of hysterical reaction enables the patient to forget or blot out an unwelcome or painful experience, such as a car crash, through loss of memory (amnesia).

An *obsessional* or *compulsive neurosis* occurs when a person has continually bizarre ideas that may seriously interrupt normal mental activity. The patient feels almost possessed by these ideas; he feels they may take over his brain completely. Repetitive thoughts may be reflected in repetitive actions. A person may have to return to his house several times to make sure he has shut the door or turned off all the lights. Unless he chooses to tell someone or seek advice, such an individual may suffer considerable mental anguish for years without anybody else being aware of it.

A *depressive reaction* or *neurosis* is related to the loss of someone or something important—a broken love affair, bereavement, retirement, a thwarted ambition. It is an acute form of withdrawal from a conflict that causes guilt, despair, and sometimes suicide.

If stress causes a breakdown and a mental disorder that affects you or a lover or close relative or friend, seek help without delay. You should see a doctor as soon as possible if you or someone close to you have a compulsion or have tried to commit suicide or attack somebody; if you are severely depressed or in despair; or if you have severe mental disturbances, such as delusions, hallucinations, or bizarre ideas. You also should see your doctor if your depression, nervousness, tension, or other mental disturbance is severe enough to interfere with your work; if insomnia lasts more than four nights; if you have bouts of undue nervousness, irritability, aggressiveness, or weeping; if your behavior is abnormal in terms of truancy, deception, or dishonesty; if you have irrational or inappropriate ideas or reactions or serious worries about work or school, family or marriage, social or sexual relationships, money, or housing; if you excessively consume alcohol or drugs; or if you have a phobic or hysterical disorder.

Many breakdowns and neuroses, especially the anxious and depressive types, can be effectively and quickly treated once a diagnosis of the illness and its cause has been made. Most patients do not have to be hospitalized for treatment, and some do not have to miss work. Psychological tests may be necessary to establish the patient's basic personality type. But the patient's first need is to be able to talk to the doctor about what has been going wrong and how he feels. Gradually the doctor and the patient explore the meaning of the patient's symptoms and the reasons for them. They continue this exploration until the real trouble is out in the open and the patient can release his associated feelings of shame or anger, sadness or resentment.

Doctor and patient then can consider what to do about the problem. Treatment may involve changing the way the patient spends his time or money, or it may involve changing the direction of the patient's life. The patient may have to learn to stand up to a bullying boss or a domineering spouse. This treatment, in which the patient does most of the talking while the therapist gently leads the direction of the monologue, is called psychotherapy. A psychotherapist may be a doctor who specializes in mental disorders (psychiatrist), or he may be the patient's general practitioner, a psychotherapist who is not a doctor, or a specially trained social worker.

There are many "schools" of psychotherapy, and each holds different beliefs about how the mind works. One form of psychotherapy, based on the teachings of Sigmund Freud, is called psychoanalysis. Psychoanalysis involves bringing into the open the desires and conflicts that have been forced into the subconscious mind and later expressed in a mental disorder. Group psychotherapy relies on the open exchange of information about and frank discussion of each member's problems under the leadership of a psychiatrist or psychotherapist. Behavior therapy tries to change a patient's actions by providing disagreeable responses to his abnormal behavior and associating pleasant responses with more normal reactions. Just as you would not take powerful drugs or have an operation unless a doctor ordered them for you, so you should not undergo any form of psychotherapy without seeking medical advice first.

The doctor may also consider drug therapy. He may prescribe a sedative or sleeping tablet (hypnotic) for a time to ensure adequate rest or tranquilizing or antianxiety drugs to control tension. Some of the common ones are diazepam (Valium), lorazepam (Ativan), and chlordiazepoxide (Librium). All of these drugs are to some extent sedative; so they should not be taken with alcohol or when driving. They can be addictive and therefore should not be taken longer than strictly necessary. Monoamine oxidase inhibitor drugs may be used to treat patients with a phobia or an obsessive or depressive neurosis. Great care must be taken with these drugs. Monoamine oxidase inhibitors interact with many drugs.

They also interact with cheese, meat extracts, beans, and alcohol, and they may produce a severe reaction.

Hospitalization may be necessary, especially if the patient is a danger to himself or others; if his disturbance is more than his family can cope with; or if he needs continuous observation or treatment. The patient will spend the first few days getting complete rest. The hospital staff will make sure all his needs are met, and they will give him whatever drugs are necessary. As the patient's strength and confidence return, he will be encouraged to take more responsibility for himself. He will engage in psychotherapy, probably involving individual interviews and group therapy, and possibly occupational, art, and drama therapy as well. The goal of such care is to build up the patient's self-confidence so he can begin making decisions and accepting responsibilities. He will have trial periods at home, and, when ready, he will be discharged from the hospital. Afterward, he will be followed up individually by his doctor or by community mental health or psychiatric services.

A nervous breakdown is an "acute" illness, like appendicitis or pneumonia, and the likelihood of complete recovery is high. Complications, unpleasant aftereffects, and later trouble can occur. But most people return to full, healthy lives and bear only the memory of their illness.

EXERCISE IS ESSENTIAL

Even though dieting and avoiding smoking and stress are the most important factors in "staying on top," adequate exercise also is essential to good health and maximum fitness. In an age when most of us get little or no regular exercise (we drive to work, sit down all day, drive home, and sit down all evening) we must make an effort to get as much of it as we need.

Your body thrives on being used. Without sufficient exercise, the unused parts, particularly the muscles, joints, lungs, and blood vessels, begin to deteriorate and become considerably less efficient than they could be. Your body as a whole loses its edge over disease and its feeling of fitness. With sufficient exercise, however, your muscles and joints become stronger and more resistant to strain. Your lungs and breathing capacity increase. The circulation in your blood vessels and heart improves, reducing the chance of a heart attack. The extra use of energy helps keep you slim. The activity as an outlet for frustration and aggression makes you more relaxed.

The type of exercise you choose is important. To be effective, exercise must be vigorous. You should engage in keep-fit exercises—running or jogging, tennis or squash, swimming, hill climbing, or heavy gardening. Walking, golf, dancing, and light gardening are better than nothing, but not much. The exercise should involve movement (it should be dynamic) as opposed to straining against an immovable object, such as pushing a broken-down car, since static exercise may be harmful. You must work up to a level of exertion that causes sweating and mild breathlessness. And you must exercise for at least thirty minutes three times a week. Excessive exercise, especially when trying to do too much too quickly, can be dangerous; so consult your doctor if you have been out of condition for some time and are contemplating taking up a strenuous sport. Also take your time and gradually work up to strenuous activity through a proper training program.

The program of exercises presented in the Appendix (see page 205) was designed by Al Murray, Great Britain's National and Olympic Coaching Adviser, in conjunction with the Health Education Council of Great Britain. The program is safe and effective, suitable for almost everybody, and takes no more than fifteen to twenty minutes three times a week. It is progressive and complete; it gradually increases the level of exertion and ensures that every part of the body is exercised. The program involves three groups of exercises. The first—mobility exercises—puts the main joints and muscles through their full range of movements. The second—strengthening exercises—works against resistance to enhance strength for specific occasions that require effort, such as running for a bus, making a long climb, or lifting a heavy weight. The third—heart and lung exercises—gives you greater efficiency and reserve power in the respiratory and circulatory systems. You cannot be too fit; so for those who want more than the basic requirement, there also is a set of more advanced training exercises.

Many forms of exercise will help keep you fit, but each varies in what it can offer in terms of stamina, suppleness, and strength. Here are the advantages of common sports and other activities.

There are a great many other forms of exercise that will contribute to keeping you fit, though they each vary in precisely what they can offer you in terms of stamina, suppleness, and strength. Here is a "league table" of various common sporting and other activities.

Key

★ No real effect	★★★ Very good effect
★★ Beneficial effect	★★★★ Excellent effect

	Stamina	Suppleness	Strength
Badminton	★★	★★★	★★
Canoeing	★★★	★★	★★★
Climbing stairs	★★★	★	★★
Cycling (hard)	★★★★	★★	★★★
Dancing (ballroom)	★	★★★	★
Dancing (disco)	★★★	★★★★	★
Digging (garden)	★★★	★★	★★★★
Football	★★★	★★★	★★★
Golf	★	★★	★
Gymnastics	★★	★★★★	★★★
Hiking	★★★	★	★★
Housework (moderate)	★	★★	★
Jogging	★★★★	★★	★★
Judo	★★	★★★★	★★
Mowing lawn by hand	★★	★	★★★

	Stamina	Suppleness	Strength
Rowing	★★★★	★★	★★★★
Sailing	★	★★	★★
Squash	★★★	★★★	★★
Swimming (hard)	★★★★	★★★★	★★★★
Tennis	★★	★★★	★★
Walking (briskly)	★★	★	★
Weight lifting	★	★	★★★★
Yoga	★	★★★★	★

Regardless of the sport you choose, you will get real benefit from it only if you do it regularly—at least two or three times a week. Go easy to start with and work up to full exercise pitch gradually. And don't expect miracles. It takes about six weeks before you really feel the benefit. Often the biggest difficulty is getting started at all. You may not like the idea in the first place and may be too busy to find the time anyway.

So while you're thinking about what you can't do, try taking a walk, then another and another. Almost before you realize it, you'll be taking the first steps back to fitness. If you're over age 35 and out of condition, walking is the most comfortable and the safest way of getting back into shape. Try walking at least part of the way to work. Walk to do the shopping. Walk in the park at lunchtime. And don't dawdle. Stride out briskly and confidently. Just take longer, faster paces, and swing the rest of your body loosely and naturally in rhythm. Sustained walks of ten minutes or more once, then two or three times a day, will soon help build up your stamina.

And take to the hills whenever you can. You'll find it well worth the effort and excellent for building up stamina. But if the hills are high or you're going far, take plenty of wool garments and a waterproof coat to keep yourself warm and dry. Study the map, stick to the paths, and make sure you return before dusk.

You don't have to brave the elements to exercise. You can

keep fit indoors. Walk up the stairs instead of riding the elevator or escalator; five minutes a day of concentrated stair-climbing can really keep your heart and lungs toned up. Five minutes of dancing a day, ten minutes every other day, or fifteen to twenty minutes three times a week will soon shake you into shape. Try to avoid those smoky discotheques where the music is too loud and there isn't room to move. You may find a local dance class more to your liking.

Jogging

Jogging is a particularly good form of exercise. It not only makes you feel great, it also is one of the most natural and effective ways of exercising the heart and lungs. Jogging is running free and easy at a comfortable trot. There's no urgency, no strain, no competition.

The idea is to jog at a pace that makes you moderately breathless. If you jog long enough and often enough in gradually increasing sessions (see below), you soon will build up the stamina of your heart and lungs and strengthen your leg muscles. And the steady, easy rhythm of jogging will help massage away mental and physical tension and lift depression. The beauty of jogging is that virtually anyone can do it. You can do it, anywhere and anytime.

The best time of day to jog is when it suits you: before breakfast when the air is fresh and the streets are quiet, in the evening before supper or under cover of darkness. When you jog depends on how you feel and how your day is planned. But there are times when you should *not* jog:

- Don't jog within two hours of your last meal.
- Don't jog if you feel tired or weak.
- Don't jog if you have a cold or feel one coming on.
- Don't jog in fog.

When you do jog, make yourself comfortable; wear loose-fitting lightweight clothing. Natural fibers, such as cotton, are preferable to synthetics because they keep you cool. You want to stay cool so you won't become quickly exhausted. But if you're too cold, your muscles may stiffen into a cramp. So wear a warm top that you can take off and sling around your waist when you start to warm up. A track suit is tailor-made for the job. In cold weather, keep your head warm by wearing a hat or scarf. And, remember, if you jog in the dark, always wear light-colored clothing so you can be seen by fast-moving traffic. Even better, wear a reflective jacket.

Also be sure to wear the proper footgear. If you have an old pair of gym shoes that are broken in but haven't broken up, wear them. If you're buying a new pair, keep these points in mind:

- Choose shoes that have a thick cushioned rubber insole, especially at the heel. The cushioned insole prevents jarring.
- Watch out for protruding stitches on the inside; they might cause blisters.
- Avoid shoes with plastic linings that don't let your feet "breathe."
- Avoid shoes with high tabs at the back; they may cut into your heel.
- Choose a shoe with good arch support.
- Choose a size larger than your street shoes if you intend to wear thicker socks since your feet may "spread" a little while jogging.
- Break in new shoes by wearing them in the house for a few days before you jog with them.

As with any other heart and lung exercise, you will get the most benefit by jogging as often as possible, preferably every day. But if you can't manage that, jog every other day. Less often and you lose the training effect.

How much you jog depends on your state of fitness. The most important thing is to build up your jogging gradually week by week. This build-up gives your heart, lungs, and circulation time to develop stamina. On the following pages are two different build-up schedules—one for someone under age 35 or someone over that age who is reasonably fit and one for those over 35 or those who are unfit. Eventually you should jog at least ten (preferably twenty) minutes each session.

Start jogging gently, especially if you are over age 35, unfit, overweight, or smoke. Here's how to build up your effort gradually day by day. You should always be well within your capability. If you feel "burned out," you've overdone it.

Build-Up Schedule A

For fairly fit people under 35 years of age.

Week 1—Briskly walk for a half-hour a day. Walk at every opportunity: use the stairs, get off the bus a stop or two earlier, walk to do the shopping. Walk briskly during the entire daily jogging session.

Week 2—Start by walking for five minutes. Jog for thirty seconds and walk for thirty seconds. Repeat ten times. Jog for forty-five seconds and walk for forty-five seconds. Repeat three times. Walk five minutes.

Week 3—Walk five minutes. Jog one minute and walk one minute. Repeat five times. Walk five minutes.

Week 4—Walk two minutes. Jog two minutes and walk one minute. Repeat five times. Walk two minutes.

Week 5 and thereafter—Walk one minute. Jog three minutes and walk one minute. Repeat five times. Over the next few weeks, increase the time spent jogging and cut down the number of walking breaks until you are jogging for twenty minutes.

Build-Up Schedule B

For not-so-fit people over 35 years of age.

Week 1—Spend a week walking as much as possible as described in Schedule A. Work up to a half-hour of brisk walking a day.

Week 2—Start by walking for five minutes. Jog fifteen seconds and walk fifteen seconds. Repeat five times. Walk five minutes. Jog fifteen seconds and walk fifteen seconds. Repeat five times. Walk five minutes.

Week 3—Walk five minutes. Jog thirty seconds and walk thirty seconds. Repeat three times. Walk four minutes. Jog ten seconds and walk thirty seconds. Repeat three times. Walk five minutes.

Week 4—Walk five minutes. Jog one minute and walk one minute. Repeat twice. Walk two minutes. Jog one minute and walk one minute. Repeat twice. Walk five minutes.

Week 5—Walk five minutes. Jog one minute and walk one minute. Repeat five times. Walk five minutes.

Week 6—Walk two minutes. Jog two minutes and walk one minute. Repeat five times. Walk two minutes.

Weeks 7 and 8—Gradually increase the time spent jogging and cut down the number of walking breaks until, by the end of the eighth week, you are jogging for ten to twenty minutes at a stretch.

Poise and Relaxation

Poise and relaxation also help keep you fit. They minimize physical and mental stress. We must give special attention to poise and relaxation because physical exertion diminishes as modern mechanical contrivances increase. Poise or the way we stand and move and a physically and mentally relaxed attitude toward our surroundings and what happens to us are vital if we are to avoid the stress associated with modern living.

To understand the importance of posture, we must consider the human machine. Man's normal standing posture has taken millions of years to evolve, and the evolution is repeated with each baby as he progresses from being a four-legged creature who crawls on his hands and knees to a two-legged creature who stands and walks. After being curled up in his mother's womb for nine months, the infant needs time to straighten out his legs and spine. By the age of twelve or fifteen months, the infant is strong enough and sufficiently well balanced to stand upright.

The overwhelming physical force to which the human machine is exposed is gravity. By maintaining an erect posture, we constantly challenge this force. The body's center of gravity and its functional focus, the point at which the weight is balanced, is in the pelvis (see figure A, page 176). Since all activities of the standing body rely on the pelvis, it is the part of the skeleton that is most sensitive to stress and injury. With good posture and good muscle control, the pelvis will not be exposed to dangerous stresses.

The body's movements are controlled by muscles, which constrict to move the bony levers of the skeleton. Effective body movement depends on the action and relaxation of opposing muscles. Man's erect posture is achieved by a fine adjustment of muscular action concentrated in the pelvis, and it is reinforced by the support and assistance of the related ligaments (see figure B). Poor posture adversely affects the internal organs and often causes faulty digestive and bowel function and poor chest expansion. Economic muscular effort and precise muscle control improve when stress and anxiety are absent.

Good posture is largely a matter of keeping good muscle tone and rhythm and balance between all the postural muscles throughout the body. We must make a conscious effort to maintain proper posture and to keep all the muscles and joints in good condition. In this example of poor posture (figure C, page 176), the spine curves in, the stomach bulges forward, and the bosom droops. It's unattractive and harmful as well. By correcting her posture, the girl will improve her appearance and her health. She also will feel more alert at the end of the day. Poor posture and poor relaxation often contribute to accidents at home, in the factory or office, and on the streets.

Backache is one of the most common causes of pain and absence from work. It usually is due to excessive stress placed on the body's center of gravity by improperly lifting heavy

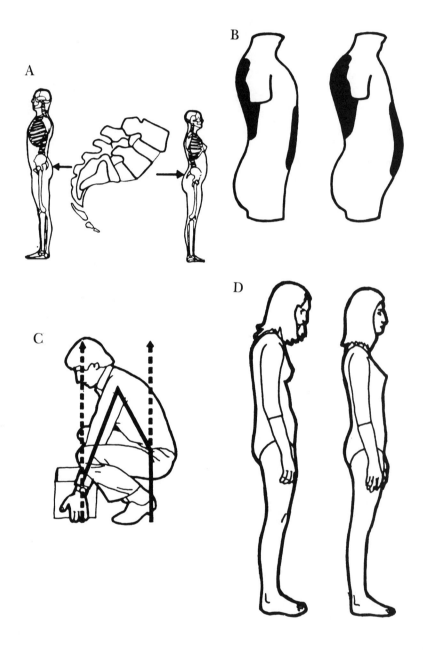

objects. When people lift objects by bending over at the hips and keeping the knees straight, they increase the effect of the weight by two or three times. They also place all the strain of the weight on the ligaments, which become stretched. Heavy weights should be lifted in this way (figure D). This method of lifting does not put the back under strain because all the available joints and muscles are being used.

To ensure correct posture and avoid strains and accidents, posture training is necessary. This training should be part of children's general physical education. It can be fun and can help youngsters learn how their body works. Good posture is attractive. If you have good posture and feel good, you will look good to others.

Here are some simple exercises. Complete every action slowly and keep your full attention on it. First lie on your back on the floor or on the bed and concentrate on your breathing. Now practice complete relaxation. Focus on each part of the body. Start with the toes and work up. Let each part of the body become loose and feel it doing so. Feel your breathing become quieter and deeper and rest for several minutes. If you feel any tension or fatigue while doing the exercises that follow, return to this relaxation position for a few minutes before going on.

Now practice active deep breathing. Slowly fill your chest with as much air as you can and then exhale deeply. When breathing in, flatten the stomach muscles. When breathing out, let the stomach muscles relax. If you can't expand the chest and flatten the abdomen at first, practice flattening the stomach alone.

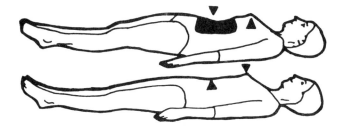

Alternately tighten and relax the muscles of the buttocks. As you move these muscles, you should notice an appreciable rise of the hip bones.

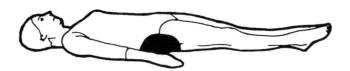

After a minute's rest, alternately raise each leg. Keep the knee straight. Repeat three or four times and rest.

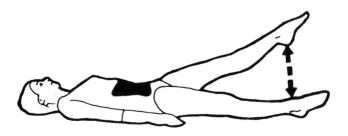

When you feel strong enough to do it without strain, raise both legs together.

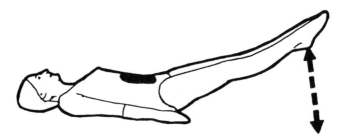

Turn over and practice straight-leg raising from this position. First lift each leg singly and then lift both together.

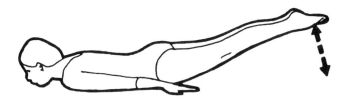

Poise and relaxation are important to health and happiness for many reasons. As you can see, the housewife on the left looks awkward and is really struggling with that heavy basket. She also is upsetting the workings of her muscles. Split in two, heavy loads can be carried comfortably. The weight on each side gives the necessary balance. The housewife on the right looks more attractive. She won't be worn out by the time she gets home, and she won't have strained her shoulder.

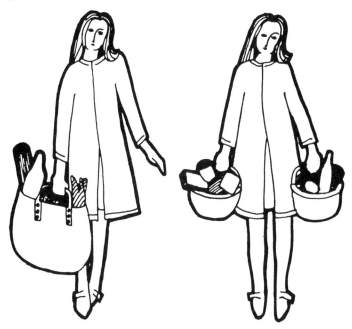

HEALTH CHECKS

Is it worthwhile to get your health checked, overhauled, and serviced at regular intervals? It is true that you may drop dead on your way home after a physical examination found nothing wrong with you because some serious conditions cannot be detected by routine health screening. It also is true that doctors cannot agree on the value of periodic health examinations. Some doctors feel that even if nothing is done about abnormalities found during a routine physical, the person will not develop disease. On the other hand, there is no doubt that regular health screening does pick up unsuspected conditions that require treatment and that otherwise may progress to an incurable state before symptoms occur. Since health checks can and do save lives, they are worthwhile. Health checks are not, and never can be, a guarantee that there is nothing wrong, however.

Regular checks of the eyes, ears, teeth, weight, heart and circulation (including the blood pressure), lungs and respiration, urine and blood, and breasts and pelvic organs in women are most important. They should be combined with a general physical examination, a determination of your own previous medical history and your family's history, and an assessment of anything that happens to be wrong with you. The ideal person to do a health check is your family doctor. He has long-term personal knowledge of your background in terms of personality, occupation, and family situation and can put physical findings into perspective. He can, therefore, give you sound advice about what changes, if any, should be made in your life. Health checks should be carried out routinely during the school years. Afterward, they should be done every five years until the age of 45 and every one or two years after that age.

THE RIGHT BALANCE

Probably the most important key to health and happiness is

obtaining the right balance between the needs of our bodies and minds and their sometimes conflicting demands. The aim should be to add life to years, not to add years to life. And to achieve the right balance, compromise in some part of our lives probably will be necessary. As far as your body is concerned, the golden rules are to:

- Eat adequate amounts of food (three well-balanced meals a day but nothing in between)
- Get adequate exercise
- Get enough sleep (between seven and eight hours a night for most people)
- Take adequate leisure and vacation time
- Drink alcohol in moderation only
- Don't smoke

Certainly no less vital to our health in the broadest sense is the balance and blend of work and leisure, risk and fulfillment, individuality and conformity, personal pleasure and family or social responsibility.

9.
Avoiding Trouble

Accidents are a common cause of death and disability, and they are on the increase. The most likely place in which accidents occur is the home.

AT HOME

Your home is a surprisingly dangerous place. Those at greatest risk of accidents in the home are children, especially infants and toddlers. But housewives and the elderly also are in danger. The greatest hazards are from cuts, electricity, fumes, poisons, fires, and falls.

Cuts. Sharp objects left lying around, broken glass, or falls through glass doors and windows are the usual causes of cuts. To avoid them, don't leave knives, tools, or razor blades out in the open. Don't use a sharp tool with the blade pointing toward you and don't try to catch a tool or knife while it is falling. Always sweep up broken glass and dispose of broken bottles and china immediately. If you have glass doors or large windows, mark them in some way (perhaps by sticking something on the panes so strangers realize what they are). Make sure glass doors and windows are well illuminated and remove nearby objects that people can slip on or trip over, such as the edge of a carpet or a doormat.

Electricity. Touching faulty wiring or exposed wires or sockets and tampering with electrical apparatus while still "live" frequently cause accidents. Check for bare wires in an electric socket and have them repaired. Don't use a damaged plug. Put dummy plugs in any socket that a crawling baby can reach with his fingers. Don't dismantle electrical apparatus or take the back off a radio or television set while the electricity is on. Don't cut electrical wires without making sure that they are "dead." Don't let wires, plugs, or electrical appliances get near water. In particular, don't switch on an electrical device with wet hands or take an appliance into the bathroom. Don't let extension cords trail along the floor or run under a carpet. Don't install new wiring in your home unless you really know what you are doing. Make sure that wires are connected properly and securely and that fuses are fitted properly.

Fumes. Leaking glass appliances or strong cleaning fluids may elicit toxic fumes. Make sure that gas stoves, boilers, water heaters, etc., are properly ventilated but don't try to service them yourself. Don't run the engine of your car in a closed garage. Don't work with glues or paints, etc., in a confined space and don't mix household cleansers together.

Choking and suffocation. Plastic bags, beads, coins, and food may suffocate or choke children. Never leave polyethylene bags lying around. Make sure that toys are safe; remove loose items or items that can be pulled or bitten off. Cut children's food small enough so they have no difficulty swallowing it. Never leave beads, buttons, or small change where young children can reach them.

Poisons. Poisoning from medicines and household chemicals is a major cause of accidental death in children. Store all medicines where children can't get at them, preferably in a locked medicine cabinet, and purchase all drugs in child-resistant containers. Don't take your own tablets or medicine in front of children; they may get ideas. Don't store disinfectants or bleaches under the kitchen sink, and don't keep household chemicals or cleaning materials in the same cupboard as food. To protect yourself, don't take anybody else's medicine. Return to your pharmacist or destroy medicines that you have finished using. Don't transfer medicines from one bottle to another or take medicine from an unlabeled bottle. Always check the label before taking a medicine.

Aerosol containers. Aerosol containers may explode; so don't put them on or near an oven or radiator or throw them on a fire. And don't spray near a fire or hot plate. Don't leave aerosols where children can get at them. The spray may damage their eyes or skin.

Fires. Fires and the burns they produce are a common cause of injury. Keep fireplaces guarded. Don't keep papers or toys on the mantelpiece or a rug in front of the fireplace. Make sure your children's clothes are made of nonflammable material. Treat electric blankets with great caution. Don't smoke in bed. Always disconnect the television when you have finished watching it. Take great care that all matches and cigarette butts are completely extinguished; don't drop them into a wastepaper basket. Don't leave matches where children can reach them. Don't dry clothes close to an open fire. Keep a fire extinguisher on each floor of your house and get a smoke detector. (For an emergency plan in case a fire breaks out, see page 16. For management of burns, see page 37.)

Hot liquids may splatter or spill on children. Don't let children or pets play in the kitchen. Even if they don't get hurt, they may trip you and make you spill a hot liquid on yourself. Pots should be placed on the stove so their handles are turned inward.

Falls. Nearly half the accidents in the home, particularly for the elderly, are due to falls. Make sure that you do not have loose banisters or stair carpets, a frayed carpet, or highly polished floors. See that all carpets are tacked down. Don't try to carry too much up or down stairs and don't carry so much in front of you that you can't see where you are going. Don't try to balance too much on a tray. Never leave things on or near the stairs—or anywhere else where people can fall over them. In the bathroom, take special care that there is nothing that you could slip on. When standing on chairs or steps make sure that they are secure, strong enough, and not close to a window or other hazard.

Do-it-yourself work can sometimes be hazardous, especially if you are doing something at which you are not skilled, using power tools to which you are not accustomed.

The garden or front yard. Don't mow the lawn in bare feet—people have cut their toes off this way. Don't tinker with an electric mower without switching it off at the source—it can have a similar effect on your fingers. If you leave a baby in the garden, make sure that he is protected with a cat net. If you have young children, and a garden pool, make sure that it's netted over. And don't forget that the garden shed is full of delightful, but highly dangerous temptations—keep it locked or effectively bolted.

On the road. As a nation we tend to drive at least to the limit of risk that the law allows, and very often beyond that—relying on the likelihood that the police cannot be everywhere and that we stand a very good chance of not being caught. Perhaps this situation appeals to the need that most of us seem to have for an element of risk and danger in our lives, and turns the needlessly hazardous driving that most of us are guilty of, into a kind of sport. Drastic reduction of this slaughter on the roads—now one of the most serious of twentieth-century epidemics—depends not so much on tightening up traffic laws as on a widespread commitment to certain basic personal driving rules. They are:

- I will get my daily ration of danger in some other way—one that does not involve putting the lives of others at risk.
- I will not drive at all if my judgment might have been affected by: alcohol—none at all is the only really safe

limit; drugs—tranquilizers and antihistamines are the worst offenders; anger; fatigue; or illness.

● I will use my seat belt at all times.
● I will observe traffic regulations at all times, no matter how hurried I am.
● I will personally check the safety of my car once a week; I will at least check the tires, lights, brakes, and steering.

Bicyclists also make up a large proportion of today's traffic casualties. Parents should make sure that their children know the safety rules and that the bicycles have sound steering and brakes and adequate lights.

Pedestrians, particularly children, are in the greatest danger of traffic accidents. Children are impulsive. They act first and think afterward, often when it is too late. They also are easily distracted from what they originally had planned and can pay attention to only one thing at a time. So even if they know safety rules by heart, they may not be able to carry them out. Other guidelines should be followed:

● Do not let any child under age 7 cross streets unsupervised.
● Teach children to cross on straight, open sections of road. Tell them not to cross streets at a crossroads, junction, or bend. Tell them to choose a place so oncoming drivers can clearly see them and they can see the drivers.
● Make sure that children know safety rules and show them, when you cross the street together, how the rules prevent accidents. Point out situations that would have resulted in an accident if people had not been careful. Follow safety rules yourself. To make an impression on them, children must see the rules in practice.

AT WORK

No type of work is free of accidents, though some jobs obviously involve more risk from moving machinery or toxic chemicals or gases. Investigation of industrial accidents shows that nearly all occur because the employer or the employee broke safety rules. So no matter how well you know the job or how hurried you are, never try to take short cuts that involve bending the safety regulations. And if it's getting toward the end of the day or you're feeling tired for some reason, doublecheck everything you do.

AT LEISURE

Leisure activities also have hazards and take a toll, particularly for those who leave their common sense at home. The greatest risk to health involves doing things which people are not accustomed to doing. Most accidents occur when people do things without adequate training and preparation or when they do things for extended periods. Every year lives are lost because people go sailing or climbing without knowing enough about what they are doing or without being sufficiently fit to cope with what is involved. Many people like to take risks and stretch themselves to the limit, but there is a world of difference between tackling a hazard for which one has prepared and a hazard that is foolhardy.

Problems that can arise from exposure to prolonged cold, wind, or rain and what to do about them are considered on pages 52–53. Thunderstorms and lightning also can be dangerous. The safest places are inside a car or building or under the branches of a group of trees—but not up against a tree.

The countryside contains other hazards. Every year hundreds of people, most of them children, eat pretty, apparently harmless flowers, berries, and fungi. Some are poisonous, a few dangerously so. Unless you make sure that you and your children leave all plants alone, you must be able to tell the safe from the unsafe.

Water and swimming also call for special care. Remember, don't go swimming alone. Don't swim out into deep water. You can have just as much fun swimming along the beach. Swim in patrolled bathing areas. Don't risk swimming in areas that post "danger" or "no swimming" signs. If you do get into difficulties, raise one arm out of the water and move it slowly from side to side.

On Vacation

Food—Some people can eat anything anywhere, but you may not be able to. So take care where you eat. Check the bathroom in a restaurant before you order. If it's filthy, the kitchen will be, too. Also take care what you eat. Bugs are most likely found in water, ice, milk, shellfish, salads, reheated foods, cold buffets, ice cream, and food from stalls. Sterilize salad makings and fresh fruit whenever possible. Add salt to your food if you have been sweating excessively.

Drink—If you have any doubt about its purity, sterilize or boil water and keep it in a refrigerator. Or drink mineral water. Beware of local juices, and watch out for the ice. You might be shocked to learn what can happen to ice. And freezing doesn't kill all the germs. But make sure you drink enough fluids. You need a pint of fluid for every ten degrees of temperature every day (that's seven pints a day at 70° F and eight pints a day at 80° F).

Clothing—Cotton is best for warm climates; it absorbs more sweat than synthetic fibers. You also may take along plenty of drip-dry gear.

Sun—Too much sun too soon will ruin the rest of your holiday. You may be surprised to learn that for most people enough sun is no more than fifteen minutes on the first day, thirty on the second, and an hour on the third. After that you can double your time in the sun every day. Be sure to apply sunscreens liberally every hour or two and after swimming.

Take it easy—You're supposed to be on vacation. Don't spoil it by trying to do too much.

Vaccinations. For travel in certain countries, some vaccinations are required by international health regulations or by individual governments. Other vaccinations are not obligatory, but having them is a sensible precaution against dangerous diseases that are common in particular parts of the world. Governments' health regulations may change suddenly, however, and it is not always easy to be sure which vaccinations are required and which are not. Failure to have had a required vaccination may lead to delay and expense. You may have to get the injection on the spot or may be refused entry to a country. It is wise, therefore, to have all the vaccinations that may be required before leaving. You also will learn of any reaction to the inoculation at home instead of in a strange country.

Your doctor will complete international certificates that report when smallpox, cholera, and yellow fever inoculations were given. You also may ask the doctor to list any other vaccinations he has given you. Some international certificates must be stamped by your local board of health before they become valid. Be sure that your certificates are stamped; otherwise they may not be accepted. Remember that vaccination certificates are needed for each person; one certificate cannot cover the whole family.

Smallpox—Few countries now require a smallpox vaccination. However, one new case of the disease in any country will make vaccination mandatory. So you may as well have it done. The vaccination, which involves a light scratch on the arm, provides immediate protection for three years. If you have been vaccinated against smallpox before, you probably will not have a reaction. If not, you may have pain, swelling, and tenderness at the site of the vaccination a week after the injection. These symptoms usually last for several days. The doctor must inspect the vaccination a week after giving it to make sure that it has "taken." If there is a medical reason why you should not have a smallpox vaccination, your doctor must sign a statement to this effect, and the statement must be stamped by the local board of health.

Cholera—Vaccination against cholera is advisable if you are going to Asia, Africa, or the Mediterranean coast. Countries also may require vaccinations after an outbreak of disease. The full course of inoculation consists of two injections that are given at an interval of four weeks. Protection lasts for six months.

Yellow fever—Some countries require yellow fever vaccination if you have passed through an area in which it occurs, for instance, Africa or South America. The vaccination is a single injection, which must not be given less than three weeks before or after a smallpox vaccination. Protection begins ten days after vaccination and lasts for ten years.

Typhoid and paratyphoid—Vaccination is advised if you are traveling outside northern Europe, Canada, the United States, Australia, or New Zealand. The full course of inoculation consists of two injections within four to six weeks of each other. Protection lasts three years.

Infectious hepatitis (yellow jaundice)—This disease is a hazard in areas that have poor sanitation. Given by injection, the vaccination provides protection for approximately six months.

Poliomyelitis—Vaccination is advised for most areas outside northern Europe, Canada, the United States, Australia, and New Zealand. Given by mouth, the full course of inoculation consists of three doses at intervals of six to eight weeks and four to six months. Even if you have been vaccinated against polio in the past, you should have a booster shot before traveling in countries in which the disease occurs.

Tetanus—Vaccination is advisable before traveling in Asia, Africa, or South America. The vaccination is given by injection in three doses at intervals of six to eight weeks and six months. A booster shot should be taken before going abroad.

Malaria—Tablets that protect against the disease should be taken if you will be traveling in or through the tropics even for a brief period. These tablets also must be taken for four weeks after returning home.

Rabies—Rabies can occur in most parts of the world. In areas in which it is known to exist, avoid all contact with animals. If you are bitten or scratched by an animal, wash the wound thoroughly with soap and water and apply an antiseptic or alcohol. If there is any chance that the animal was rabid, go at once to the nearest doctor or hospital.

Your health luggage. Here's what you may need to take along:

- Sun cream or lotion
- Sunglasses
- Eyeglasses (take a spare pair in case of an accident)
- Water-sterilizing tablets or solution
- Insect repellent
- Freshening-up cloths or a cologne stick
- Deodorant
- Antidiarrhea medicine
- Antimalaria pills, if necessary
- Travel sickness pills
- "Flight fright" pills
- Small first aid kit, including scissors, tweezers, thermometer, safety pins, antiseptic cream, burn cream, indigestion tablets, laxative, aspirin or acetaminophen, packet of assorted dressings or bandages, three-inch-wide elastic bandage, cotton balls
- Personal medicines—enough to cover you for the time you will be away
- Information about any current illnesses or treatment and any serious past illnesses or operations, allergies or sensitivities, and vaccinations
- Health insurance against the risk of accident or illness that covers all risks and provides a sum sufficient to pay for medical attention in the countries you are visiting. (Your travel agent can arrange suitable insurance coverage for you. And even if health insurance is included in the cost of your trip, you may want extra coverage.)

Have a Good Trip

By air—Airports are tedious, tiring places. Give yourself plenty of time to check in, buy books or newspapers, and get through the security control without rushing. If you suffer from "flight fright," don't let it ruin your holiday because you are ashamed to talk to your doctor. He probably will be able to give you medicine to help relax you. But make sure you know how and when you are supposed to take the drug. If you get air sick, make sure you have something for that, too. And make sure you take it at the right time; the right time for taking these drugs varies. Long flights can be boring; so take enough to read. Don't kill the time by overeating. Pressurization in an aircraft dries the air; you consequently must keep up your fluid balance, but not with fizzy drinks. Wear loose fitting clothes; intestinal gases expand at high altitudes. Long periods of sitting in a limited space cramps all body systems. Get some exercise by walking up and down the cabin a few times.

On arrival, go straight to your hotel and rest before doing anything else. Don't book a theater or a dinner party for your first night. You won't really feel like it.

During East-West flights, the time changes by one hour for every fifteen degrees of longitude. Thus New York is five hours ahead of London, and if you arrive in London at 7:00 P.M., your body will be at 2:00 P.M. Your sleep, appetite, and excretion take several days to catch up with and adjust to this time change. You need about a day for every two or three hours of time difference. While your body is catching up, you may feel ill. You may want to sleep at strange times or not want to eat at usual meal times. This phenomenon is called *jet lag*, and it can be worrisome if you're not expecting it. There's nothing you can do about jet lag except to get several hours of sleep after you arrive and to avoid taxing activities for the first couple of days.

By train or bus—Take regular, adequate, light meals during a train or bus trip. Do get yourself a sleeper on a train if you can afford it. Follow the same tips for plane travel.

By car—Plan your route beforehand. Don't drive if you have taken sedatives or tranquilizers, travel sickness drugs, alcohol, or are tired or ill. Don't drive for more than three hours without a break for a stroll and perhaps a snack. Don't attempt to drive more than 300 miles a day. Share the driving over long distances. Beware of the third day of a long trip when you probably are getting tired, bored, and fed up with your passengers. Most accidents happen on the third day out.

And If You Do Get Ill, Here's What to Do

Sunburn—Liberal applications of calomine lotion are as good as anything. If you're badly burned, you may need to see a doctor.

Diarrhea—The only medicines that are effective against intestinal infections must be prescribed. Ask your doctor about them. Don't take such drugs as a preventive measure; they may not work that way and should be kept until you actually need them. Your doctor may not wish to give you medicine before you are ill. In that case, get a bottle of kaolin mixture or some similar mixture or tablets from your pharmacist. Make sure the medicine comes in a plastic bottle; you don't want to get kaolin from a broken bottle all over your clothes. If you do need to take medicine, be sure to get the dose right. The bugs will laugh at too little, and you may become ill from too much. Make sure you take the drug long enough. If the dosage is not listed on the bottle, continue taking the medicine for at least two days after the diarrhea has stopped. Drink enough fluids. You must replace what you are losing. If you feel hungry, nibble on dry toast. If there is no sign of improvement in two days or you see blood in the stools, consult a doctor.

Fever—A fever may be due to something simple, such as too much sun or the flu. But it may not be. Stay in bed, or at least indoors, and take two aspirin or acetaminophen tablets every three or four hours. If you haven't improved in two days or you develop symptoms that seem sinister, see a doctor.

Remember that you may catch something that will not develop until you are home again. If you do become ill after returning from vacation, tell your doctor where you have been. It may be a vital clue to what's wrong with you.

10.

Medical Care

Whether a patient suffers, becomes disabled, or dies depends not only on bad luck, on failing to take the steps necessary to prevent disease, or even on the severity or the curability of the disease. It also depends on the use of the facilities that medicine offers. A few years ago many diseases could not be cured; so medical care often did not make a great deal of difference to the patient's welfare. That situation has been almost completely reversed. The number of diseases that can be successfully treated has increased enormously. Now whether people come for medical investigation early and know how to make the best use of health services makes all the difference in the world to the outcome of their diseases.

How to Get the Best from Your Doctor

Your doctor is an important person in your life. There probably will be times when your life literally will be in his hands and he will be the most important person in your life. You should, therefore, take almost as much trouble in choosing him or her as you would in choosing a husband or wife and with very much the same eye for his capacity for caring and compatibility. His skill as a doctor and your confidence in him obviously is the first consideration. But your doctor will not be able to use his skill effectively unless he understands you and the things that are bothering you. Your doctor must understand and care for you as a whole person and be able to help you deal with your emotional and social problems as well as your influenza or appendicitis. For you to get the most out of what medical care can offer, you must have a good relationship with your doctor. The two of you must form a partnership, in which you trust and respect each other. Otherwise your doctor will not be able to give you what you need because you do not believe that he knows best. He also will not be able to give you as much as he would like because he knows that you do not have faith in him. If you don't feel that you can trust your doctor in any situation that might arise, you should get another doctor. Even though your lack of trust may not seem to matter at the moment, sooner or later an emergency will arise, and your lack of faith may have disastrous consequences. This works both ways, of course. Your doctor may not feel at ease or in sympathy with you. He may realize that he is not the right doctor for you and suggest that you see somebody who can deal with your problems more satisfactorily.

To find a doctor, get a list of the doctors who practice in your area from the public library or the local medical society. A doctor whose office is close by and who has the personal recommendation of neighbors may be suitable. But you cannot be sure that a particular doctor will be right for you until you meet him. So try to arrange an introductory meeting during which you and your doctor can look each other over and decide whether you can work together.

If, after you have been working with a doctor for some time, you find that you are not happy with the way your case is being managed or have a misunderstanding with your doctor, have a full and frank discussion with him as soon as possible.

Don't consult a second doctor without telling the first. To provide effective care, the second doctor should ask the first about you as a person and about the background of your case. He also should know what drugs the other doctor prescribed so he will not order drugs that may interact. If you no longer have faith in your doctor, find another; but do so in an open, straightforward way.

How your doctor's mind works. You will get the best from your doctor if you have some idea how his mind has been trained to work. But remember that your doctor is not a machine that churns out the correct diagnosis and the appropriate treatment. As a highly complex, ever-changing individual, you are never the sum of your parts or a piece of machinery whose problems are managed on the basis of a maintenance manual. You need more than a mechanic. Certainly your doctor must have adequate technical knowledge and skill; a good bedside manner is no substitute for deficiency in these areas. But he also must be an artist and a magician to appreciate and minister to your needs.

Your doctor approaches problems methodically, and you can help him understand yours by telling him what feels wrong in an orderly way. If the story is long and complicated, make a few notes beforehand so you don't become confused when you talk to your doctor.

Your doctor will first want to know about the main thing that has gone wrong. The abnormality that has made you see your doctor is what doctors call the *presenting symptom.* Tell him as much as you can about that abnormality: how long you have had it, what happened when it first appeared, how often it occurs, what happens when it occurs, what makes it worse, what makes it better. If your problem is pain, tell your doctor what sort of pain it is—a sharp, shooting pain, a constant aching pain, or a pain that builds to a peak and then fades away. Tell him how severe the pain is—enough to keep you awake, bad enough so that you have to walk around to take your mind off it, bad enough to make you want to scream.

Your doctor then will want to know about any other, perhaps less immediately important, things that have gone wrong—your *contributing* or *secondary symptoms,* such as poor appetite and loss of weight. If you have strong feelings about what you think is wrong or are worried that you may have a particular disease, now is the time to mention it. You may be incorrect, but your hunch may be important. In any case, your doctor should know what is on your mind so he can reassure you if your fears are groundless. But remember that your symptoms—what you have noticed or felt—are what your doctor must learn from you at this point. He does not need a ready-made diagnosis even if it eventually turns out to be right. He does not want to hear, "I've got bronchitis, and I need some antibiotics." He wants to hear, "I've had a cough for four days. It sometimes wakes me up at night. I'm bringing up nasty yellow phlegm. I don't feel at all well, and I can't eat."

After he has heard about your main symptoms and asked you questions about them, your doctor may ask some general questions about other aspects of your health to make sure that nothing has been overlooked. He may ask: Are you sleeping well? Do you have indigestion or trouble with your bowels? Do you have any problems with urination? Do you get short of breath? What has your weight been doing? Do you have any particular worries? What does your work involve? Have you been traveling out of the country recently? A doctor who has not treated you before also will want to know about your previous medical history and your parents' medical background. This information may have a bearing on what is happening to you now.

In minor, straightforward cases, your doctor may be able to decide what is wrong with you and what should be done simply by talking to you. But he still will need to perform a physical examination to be sure. The examination will focus on the part of the body that seems to be out of order, but it will also include a general examination. So when your doctor listens to your heart even though you are complaining only of a pain in your big toe, he has not taken leave of his senses; he is being thorough. If the physical examination does not provide all the information the doctor needs to reach a conclusion about what is wrong or if he needs to confirm his opinion, he may arrange for special tests, such as blood tests or X-rays, or send you to a specialist.

From what you have told him and what he has found by examining you and by doing special tests, your doctor usually knows where your trouble lies and what sort of problem probably is causing it. He will have two or three strong possibilities and several less likely ones. He now must determine which of the possible diagnoses or patterns of disorder most closely fits your case. By bringing together obvious facts and subtle factors, such as your personality, occupation, current stresses and strains, he arrives at a *differential diagnosis*. Even when he has double-checked the facts and satisfied himself that his diagnosis fits all of them, he does not close his mind to other possible diagnoses or to alterations in the pattern of the disorder. Disease is a dynamic process; its features are likely to change. So a diagnosis must be frequently reviewed.

Once a diagnosis of the problem has been made, the doctor's next task is to choose the pattern of treatment or management that will correct it. Here, too, he has many factors to consider. First, he must set the long-term and major objective—to cure the condition and get you back to normal— alongside the short-term objective—to relieve your symptoms as quickly as possible. Second, he must tailor the treatment to your own circumstances. For example, he may have to avoid medicine because you are allergic to it or avoid bedrest because you are a mother with two young children or your work is important to you. The forms of treatment vary. Often, time is all that is necessary; so if you have a problem for which medicine will not speed your recovery or make any other worthwhile difference, don't feel cheated when you leave your doctor's office empty-handed. You have had your doctor's skilled opinion and advice, which are crucial.

After his consideration of the diagnosis and management of your illness, your doctor will consider the outcome of long-standing and serious diseases and what the outcome may mean to you. This determination is called the *prognosis.* Your doctor will decide if the disease will abate in a few days and you will be able to return to work next Monday. He will determine how long you will be away from work or in a hospital. He will list any restrictions that you must observe and advise a change of job, if necessary.

Finally your doctor will tell you as much about the diagnosis, treatment, and prognosis as he thinks you want and need to know. Be sure you understand what he tells you, particularly what you must do. Misunderstandings all too easily arise. If your doctor has not explained enough or has not told you as much as you would like to know, now is the best time to ask, while it is fresh in both your minds.

How to Be a Good Patient

Your doctor cannot help you as much as he is able and willing to unless you make it possible for him. You need to follow a few simple, but important, general rules.

Don't hide things from your doctor. Tell your doctor everything even if you are embarrassed or ashamed. He wants to help you, not judge you. He has met many and varied surprises in his professional life. It is unlikely that he would be shocked. He also holds anything you tell him in total confidentiality. If you have a problem, for instance with alcohol or drugs or sex or crime or some abnormal behavior, your doctor must know the real and full truth. You make it difficult, if not impossible, for him to help if you say you smoke ten cigarettes a day when you smoke a hundred or drink three double Scotches a day when you drink a bottle.

Make sensible use of your doctor's time. Most doctors look after several thousand patients. To care for them efficiently so those who are in the greatest need get the most attention is difficult, and it is effected to a great extent by the reliability and sense of responsibility of the patients. Always keep your appointments or call in plenty of time if you must cancel. Your doctor always will respond to an emergency call, but don't claim that minor problems are emergencies.

Do what the doctor has told you to do. Don't leave your doctor's office until you know what the doctor wants you to do, especially about the way to take medicine, and until you have asked all your questions. And afterward, follow your treatment exactly as it was prescribed for you.

If you don't carry out the instructions that you are given, no amount of sophisticated tests and modern medicines will be of any use to you. Sadly, patients' failure to do what they have been advised is responsible for most treatment failures. If the dose or timing of prescribed drugs doesn't make sense, discuss it with your pharmacist or talk to your doctor again. If your condition changes, let your doctor know; he may have to change your treatment. But never, never change your treatment on your own or at somebody else's suggestion. You will interfere with what your doctor has planned and may end up doing far worse.

Appendix
An Exercise Program

THE STANDARD SCHEDULE

MOBILITY EXERCISES

Mobility exercises should be done at an unhurried, relaxed tempo. Increased range should be coaxed, not forced. Breathing should be free and easy, to fit the rhythm of the movement. About 10 or 12 repetitions is enough for each exercise, and there is no need to increase this number or the speed of the movement. Progress is achieved by gently increasing the range of the movement or, when you are mobile, by maintaining this level of flexibility.

1. Arm Swinging

Start: Feet wide astride, arms hanging loosely by your sides.
Movement: Raise both arms forward, upward, backward, and sideways, in a circular motion, brushing your ears with your arms as you go past.

2. Side Bends

Start: Feet wide apart, hands on hips.

Movement: Bend first to the left and then to the right, keeping the head at right angles to the trunk.

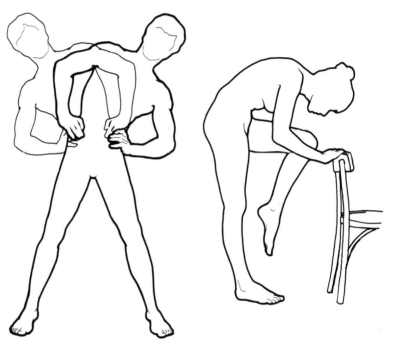

3. Trunk, Knee, and Hip Bends

Start: Stand 18 inches behind the back of a chair, with hands resting lightly on the back.

Movement: Raise the left knee and bring the forehead down to meet it. Repeat with the right knee. Do not rush. This must be a long, strong movement.

Note: When you are used to this exercise, you can dispense with the chair and work from the standing position. The supporting leg can be bent.

4. Head, Arms, and Trunk Rotating

Start: Feet wide astride, hands and arms reaching directly forward at shoulder level.

Movement: Turn the head, arms, and shoulder around to the left as far as you can go, bending the right arm across the chest; then repeat the movement to the right. Keep the hips and legs still throughout.

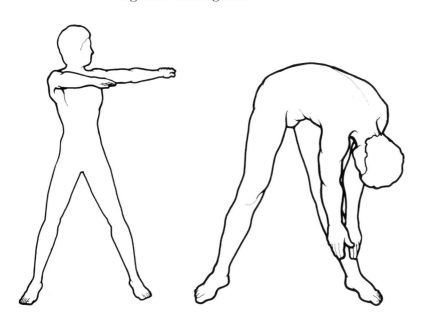

5. Alternate Ankle Reach

Start: Feet wide apart, both palms on the front of the upper left thigh.

Movement: Relax the trunk forward as you slide both hands down the front of the left leg. Return to upright position; then repeat on the right.
Note: Those suffering from mild back trouble must not pass the knees with the hands.

STRENGTH EXERCISES

1. Progressive press-ups. The standard press-up on the floor is an excellent exercise for the chest, arm, and shoulder muscles, but it is far too strenuous for unfit or overweight people. Therefore, I have split up the exercise into a series of gentle steps, as shown:

> **Stage 1:** Stand with hands on wall 12 inches apart at shoulder height, arms straight. Stand on your toes, then bend the arms until the chest and chin touch the wall. Return to starting position by straightening arms.

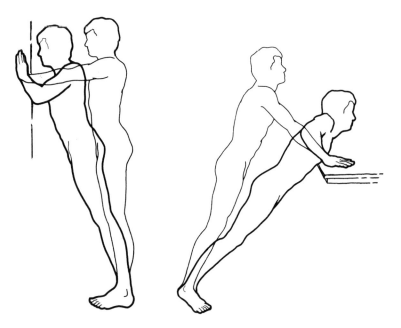

> **Stage 2:** Hands 10 or 12 inches apart on a table (be sure it is safe). Bend arms, keeping body straight, until chest touches table; then return to start position.
>
> Ladies need not progress beyond this stage.

Stage 3: As Stage 2, but using a chair. Be sure the chair is steady and that your head clears the back easily as you go down, or use two chairs.

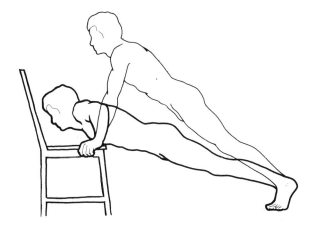

Stage 4: You should now be ready for the full press-up. Place the hands on the floor directly under the shoulders, with the fingers pointing forward. Chest and chin should touch the floor, back straight throughout.

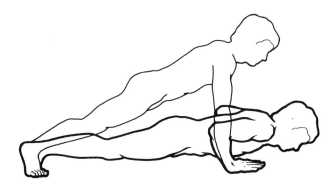

2. Abdominal exercises. These exercises, which will flatten your tummy muscles, are very worthwhile; but again the abdominal musculature can be strained if you start too enthusiastically, so the exercises are progressed.

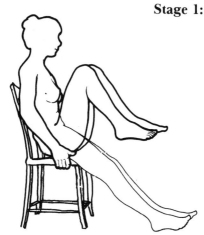

Stage 1: Sit on the front part of the chair, legs straight, heels on floor. Lean back and grip the sides of the seat for support. Bend the knees and bring the fronts of the thighs up to squeeze gently against the body.

Stage 2: Do the same exercise with the legs held straight.

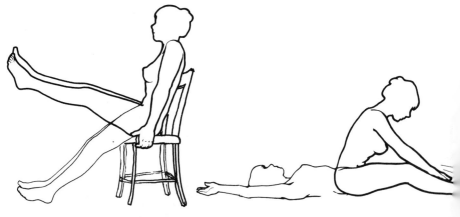

Stage 3: Lie on your back, knees slightly bent, with your feet tucked under a heavy chair or settee, arms backward stretched. Swing up to sitting position. Do not stretch any further forward than hands on ankles.

Stage 4: Lie on your back, with your hands held behind your head and your heels on the edge of a chair. Swing up to sitting position, allowing your knees to bend slightly as you do so.

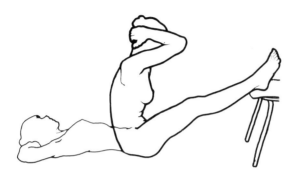

3. *Leg exercises.* These are based on squatting. As you do a squat, you will soon become aware of weakness in the legs. This is because unfit adults seldom bend their knees beyond the range needed to climb stairs or sit in a low chair.

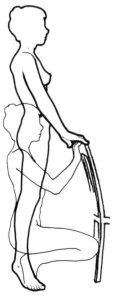

Stage 1: Stand 18 inches behind a chair, with your hands on the back. Lower the body into a squat, keeping the feet flat on the floor (ladies may stand on their toes at this point). Straighten both legs and come up on the toes, then return to the squat position.

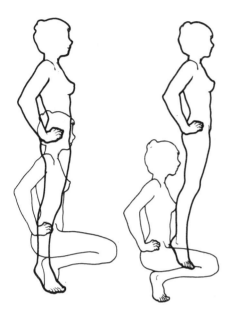

Stage 2: As in 1, but dispense with the chair and place hands on hips.

Stage 3: As in 2, but come up from the squat fast, so that your feet actually leave the floor, at first only a few inches, then a bit higher.

Stage 4: Start in the half squat position (see illustration) and leap upward into a star jump. As you land, give at the knees to take up the shock.

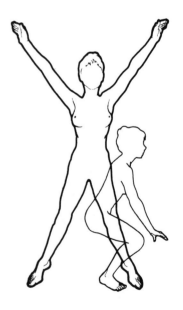

How to Use the Strength Exercises

Start at the lowest level of each exercise and do 8 to 10 repetitions of each. Gradually increase this number to 20 or 30. When you can do this comfortably, progress to the next stage of the exercise, again working up from 8 or 10 to 20 or 30, change to the next level, and so on. It is a good idea to do the leg exercises in groups of 5, resting briefly between each group. *Do not be in a hurry to progress.* Wait until you can do the full number of repetitions at one level comfortably. Heroics are not only silly, they can be dangerous.

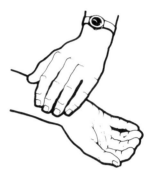

HEART AND LUNG EXERCISES

The best index of how hard the heart muscle is exercising is the pulse rate and you will have to learn how to monitor your pulse during this stage of the schedule. To take your pulse, turn the palm of the hand toward the ceiling with the wrist bared. Lightly place the first three fingers of the left hand just above the heel of the right thumb. Count off the beats on a wristwatch for 15 seconds, then multiply by four to give the rate per minute.

Broadly speaking, the speed at which the heart beats depends on the oxygen content of the blood. If the oxygen level of the blood falls, the heart beats faster. Therefore, if we exercise the large muscle groups in the trunk, arms, and legs, which use up a great deal of oxygen, this will raise the pulse rate. But how high should we raise the pulse, and for how long?

The answer to this question lies in your **personal pulse rating.** You find this by subtracting your age from 200, then subtracting a further handicap of 40 for unfitness. (This can

be reduced to about 20 as you get fitter.) So, a lady of 38 years
of age would have a personal pulse rating of

$$
\begin{array}{r}
200 \\
38 \\
\hline
162 \\
40 \quad \text{less unfitness handicap} \\
\hline
122 \quad \textbf{Personal pulse rating}
\end{array}
$$

The aim is to maintain this pulse rate and no higher for a
period of 10 minutes continuous exercise. When you do one of
the heart and lung exercises listed below, you take your pulse
rate every minute or so. If it is at, or below, your personal
pulse rating, then you continue; if above, you rest until the
pulse comes down. In unfit people, this will mean lots of
stopping and starting to begin with but with practice, the rest
periods get shorter and shorter until you can go for the whole
ten minutes without stopping, as shown in the diagram.

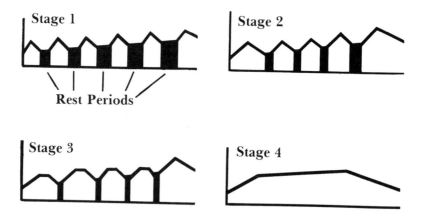

Stages 1–2—Running on the Spot

Stand with arms loosely by the sides and gently run on the spot. Do not begin by raising the knees high, but aim to get them higher as you progress. Start with a very short time—say 30 seconds—and gradually build up to 5 or 6 minutes, checking the pulse frequently.

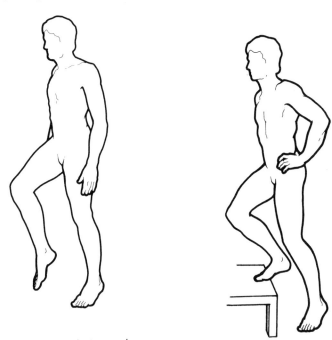

Stage 3—Bench Stepping

Take a low box or stool and stand 12 inches away from it, hands on hips. Step up onto it 15 times with the left foot leading, then 15 times with the right foot leading. Increase by 1 step per foot at each exercise session, until you are doing 30 steps with each foot. Then gradually increase the height of the bench to a maximum of 18 inches. When you can do this comfortably, start working on a time base, aiming at 3 to 6 minutes continuous exercise without exceeding your personal pulse rating.

Stage 4—Outdoor Exercise

Once you are comfortable with Stage 3, choose between jogging, swimming, or cycling and aim to do 10 minutes continuously. This will mean pauses for rest and pulse regulation as usual. After a month or two, you can cautiously raise your pulse rating by steps of 5 up to a maximum of 20. You can also improve fitness by increasing the duration of the exercise, but by this time you'll certainly be fit and "in the pink" anyway!

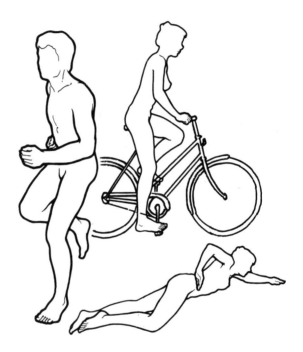

THE STANDARD SCHEDULE SUMMARIZED

Three exercise sessions per week, each lasting 15 to 20 minutes. The five mobility exercises start each session. These do not progress. Strength exercises progressed from 8 or 10 to 20 or 30 at each stage. Heart and lung exercises, pulse regulated. Do not start until rest of schedule established.

Stage 1: Press-ups against wall.
　　　　　Thigh raising seated in chair.
　　　　　Squats behind chair back.

Stage 2: Press-ups on table top.
　　　　　Straight leg raising in chair.
　　　　　Squats without a chair.
　　　　　Running on the spot.

Stage 3: Press-ups on chair seat.
　　　　　Sit-ups from lying on floor.
　　　　　Jumps from squatting position.
　　　　　Bench stepping.

Stage 4: Full press-ups on floor.
　　　　　V-sit with heels on chair.
　　　　　Star jumps.
　　　　　Jogging, cycling, or swimming.

Don't worry if you don't proceed neatly from one stage to the other in each exercise at the same time. Work at your own rate. In some exercises you may move ahead fast, others slow. Take as much time as you need.

THE ADVANCED SCHEDULE

The Advanced Schedule is based on training with weights and *you need to have completed the Standard Schedule,* and to be fit, before starting it. As with the Standard Schedule, we start off with the set of 5 mobility exercises, but in this schedule the strength and heart/lung exercises are welded together in the weight training program. It's important to realize that we are talking about weight *training,* not competitive weightlifting. The weights used are quite light—3 to 5 pounds and no more than 30 pounds maximum for the fitter person—and the accent is on repetitions rather than lifting very large loads. Heart/lung exercise is assured by gradually reducing the rest periods between exercises and making sure you keep to your personal pulse rating.

Obviously a weight training schedule is going to require weights and the best tools for the job are a barbell and a dumbbell. This will involve a modest financial outlay, but if you are going in for this program seriously, it is a small price to pay for improved physical fitness. If, on the other hand, you are waiting for Christmas or for your birthday, you can start off quite happily with a couple of plastic bottles—the sort used for liquid detergent, for instance—and fill them with water. They will then weigh around 2 pounds each. Later you can replace the water with sand, which about doubles the weight.

As with the strength exercises in the Standard Schedule, start with about 8 or 10 repetitions per exercise and build up gradually to about 20 or 30. Start with reasonable rests between each exercise and gradually reduce them as your stamina increases.

Exercises for the Advanced Schedule

Don't forget to do the mobility exercises first.

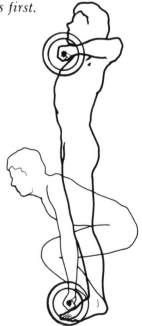

1. Chin High Pull

Insteps underneath the bar, 10 inches apart. Bend knees, look straight to the front, keep the back flat but not vertical. Grip the bar with the knuckles toward the front. Extend the body by standing up and pulling the bar in a straight line close to the body until the bar is under your chin. Complete the movement by lowering the bar to the thighs, then bending the legs back to the standing position.

2. Palms Forward Curl

Stand erect, holding the bar at arms length, palms facing forward. Flex the arms to bring the bar up to the chest; then return to start position. Keep rest of body still throughout.

3. Press Behind Neck

Stand erect, bar resting across back of neck and shoulders. Extend arms to full length above head and return.

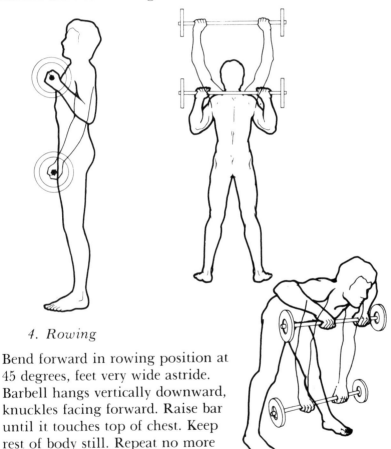

4. Rowing

Bend forward in rowing position at 45 degrees, feet very wide astride. Barbell hangs vertically downward, knuckles facing forward. Raise bar until it touches top of chest. Keep rest of body still. Repeat no more than 15 times.

5. *Side Bends*

Feet well astride, dumbbell held in left hand with right hand on hip. Bend to the left as far as you can, and then to the right. The dumbbell hangs loosely and is not involved in the effort. Do all your repetitions on one side, then change hands and repeat on the other side (*i.e.* do not keep changing from side to side).

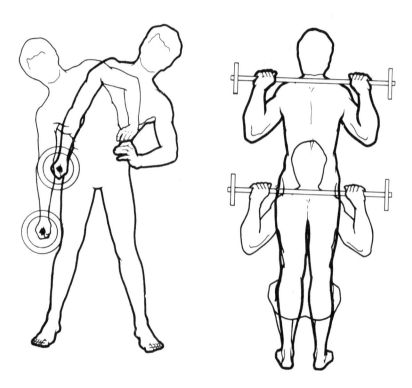

6. *Squats*

Feet about 10 inches apart, barbell behind neck on shoulders. Bend knees, keeping back straight, until the thighs are almost parallel; then come up briskly on tiptoe. Lower back to starting position, with feet flat on floor.

7. Bench Press

Lie on your back on a firm support, knees flexed. Barbell resting on chest, palms forward. Extend arms to full length and lower again.

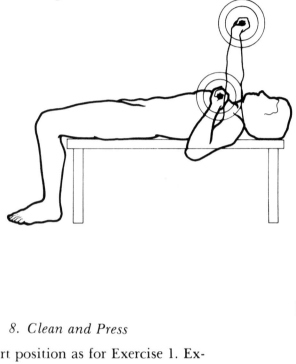

8. Clean and Press

Start position as for Exercise 1. Extend body and pull bar straight up close to the body, until it rests on the top of the chest. Then press bar overhead to arm's length. Lower bar to chest and then thighs and bend legs and lower into starting position.

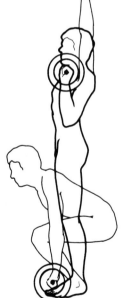

9. Sit-Ups

This exercise does not use weights, but is the correct thing to do at this place in the schedule. Start with the sit-ups described in Stage 4 of the abdominal strengthening exercises in the Standard Schedule and when you can do those comfortably progress to V-sits. Lie on back, with arms outstretched behind head. Raise legs, trunk, and arms at same time to balance on hips, reaching forward as if trying to grasp ankles. Return to lying position.

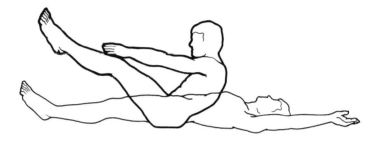

10. Straight Arm Pullover

This is a quieting-down exercise, and a very light weight should be used because of leverage. Lie on back on bench, as in Exercise 7, bar across front of thighs, palms downward. Raise bar back to behind head, keeping arms straight throughout the range of movement. Return to resting position.

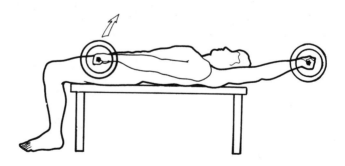

Index

A

Abdominal exercises, 210–11
Abdominal injuries, 70–71
Abdominal pain, 79–80
Abdominal thrust, 32
Accidents, 139
  plan for, 15–16
  prevention of, 183–89
  as top killer, 137
Acetaminophen, 9, 10, 31, 60, 64, 65, 84
Acetylsalicylic acid, 9
Aching. See Pain
Aerosol containers, and accident prevention, 185
Air travel, 193
Alcohol consumption, and hangovers, 60
Alcoholism, 137, 139
Alternate ankle reach, 207
Amenorrhea, 73
Anemia, 85
Anorectics, 151
Anorexia, 21–22
Antacids, 9
Antidiarrhea mixture, 9–10

Antiseptics, 10
Anus, 20–21, 29
  bleeding from, 20, 29
  discharge, 20
  itching, 20
  lumps, 20
  pain, 20
  ulcers of, 96–97
Anxiety. See Emotional disorders
Anxiety neurosis, 163
Appendicitis, 79–80
Appetite
  too little, 21–22
  too much, 22
Arm, fractures of, 71–72
Arm swinging, 205
Asphyxia, 31
Aspirin, 9, 10, 31, 65, 84
Aspirin gargle, 92
Athlete's foot, 73
Ativan, 166

B

Back, pain of, 80–81, 176–77

Bandages, 109–10
Barium
  enema, 21, 39
  swallow, 63
Bed
  care of patient in, 112–13
  comfort in, 114–16
  making of bed with patient in,
    113–14
Behavior therapy, 166
Bench press, 221
Bench stepping, 215–16
Bereaved person, care of, 124–25
Bicycling, and accident prevention,
  187
Bites, treatment of, 22–25
Black-eye, 56
Bleeding
  from anus or rectum, 20, 29
  from ears, 26–27
  from mouth, 27–29
  from nose, 27
  from vagina, 29
  from wounds, 25–26
  stopping severe, 14
  in urine, 29
Blisters, 30
Boils, 30–31
Breathing
  and Holger-Nielsen method of
    resuscitation, 33–34, 48
  lack of, 14
  and mouth-to-mouth
    resuscitation, 31–33
  and pain, 34–35
  shortness in, 35–36
  and Silvester method, 34
  stopped, 31
Bronchitis, 41, 137, 139, 154
Bruising, 36
Burns, 36–38, 50
  prevention of, 185
  treatment of, 14
Bus travel, 193

C

Calamine lotion, 10, 38, 73,

Cancer, 45, 80, 137, 139
Car travel, 194
Cardiac compression, 33
Cast, care of patient in, 119
Castor oil cream, 10, 21
Check-ups, getting regular, 180–81
Chemical burns, 37–38
  in the eye, 55
Chest
  injuries to, 70
  pain of, 81–83
Chilblain, 73
Childbirth, 29
  care of patient after, 119–20
Children
  accidental death of, 7–8
  care of sick, 117–19
  medicines for, 10
  with diarrhea, 46
Chills, 38
Chin high pull, 218
Chlor-Trimeton, 11
Chlordiazepoxide, 166
Chlorhexidine Hibiclens, 108
Choking, 31, 38
  prevention of, 184
Cholecystogram, 63
Cholera vaccination, 190–91
Chronic nasal inflammation, 11
Chronically ill person, care of, 121–
  22
Clean and press, 221
Cold compress, 110
Colitis, 20
Collar bone, fractured, 70–71
Colon, cancer of, 45
Colostomy, care of patient after, 120
Coma, 38, 97–98
Compulsive neurosis, 164
Constipation, 38–40
  treatment of, 11
Convulsions, 40–41, 46
Coping mechanisms, 162
Cough, treatment of, 10, 41–43
Cramps, 43
Crushing injuries, 67
  first aid for, 67–68
Cuts

prevention of, 183–84
See also Bleeding; Wounds

D

D & C (dilation and curettage), 74
Deafness, 44–45
Death
  care of person facing, 122–24
  most common killing diseases, 137
Depression. *See* Emotional disorders
Depressive reaction, 165
Dermatitis, 73
Diabetes, 22, 99
Diarrhea, 194
  treatment of, 9–10, 45–46
Diazepam, 166
Differential diagnosis, 201
disabled person, care of, 121–22
Disc, injuries to, 80
Discharges
  anal, 20
  ear, 49
  urethral, 98–99
  vaginal, 100–101
Dislocations, 67
Diuretics, 151
Dizziness, 46–47
  first aid for, 47–48
Do-it-yourself activities, and accident prevention, 186–87
Doctor
  deciding whether or not to see, 1–4, 19–20
  getting best care possible from, 197–203
  obtaining medical help from, 117–18
Donnegal, 9
Dressings, 105, 109
Drowning, 48
Drug therapy, 166
Drugs, for the overweight, 151
Dying. *See* Death
Dysentery, 20, 45
Dysmenorrhea, 73
Dyspareunia, 83
Dyspepsia, 62–63, 159

Dysphagia, 93
Dyspnea, 35–36
Dysuria, 99

E

Ears
  bleeding from, 26–27
  and deafness, 44–45
  discharge, 49
  foreign body, 50
  preparations for, 11
Eczema, 72
Electrical accidents, 50
  prevention of, 184
Emergency phone numbers, 7
Emotional disorders, 51–52
  care of person with, 120–21
Endemic, 137
Ephedrine, 11, 76
Epidemics, 137
Epistaxis, 27
Epsom salts, 40
Esophagitis, 93
Exercise, 150, 167–74, 205–22
  advanced schedule in, 217–22
  benefits of, 167–71
  heart and lung, 213–17
  and jogging, 171–74
  mobility, 205–7
  and poise and relaxation, 174–79
  strength, 208–23
Exposure, 38, 52–53
Eyes
  black, 56
  chemicals in, 55
  foreign body in, 55–56
  preparations for, 11
  problems of, 53–54
  wounds to, 55

F

Face, pain of, 83
Fainting. *See* Dizziness
Falls, prevention of, 185–86
Fatigue, 56–57, 85
Fibrositis, 34, 64, 82

Fire
  plan for, 16–17
  prevention of, 185
First aid, plan for, 13–15
Fish hook injuries, 57
Flushing, 57–58
Food poisoning, 45
Foods, caloric value of common,
  144–48
Foot, fractures of, 72
Foreign bodies, 58–59
  in ear, 50
  in eye, 55–56
  fish hooks as, 57
  in nose, 75
  removal from wound, 25
  splinters as, 92–93
Fractures
  of arm, 71–72
  and care of patient in a cast, 119
  of collar bone, 70–71
  crushing injuries, 67–68
  dislocations, 67
  first aid for, 67
  of jaw, 69
  of leg or foot, 72
Freud, Sigmund, 166

G

Gall bladder, disease of, 63, 79
Gargles, 10
Gastroenteritis, 45, 46
Genitals, ulcers of, 96–97
Giddiness. See Dizziness
Gingivitis, 27
Glands, 59–60
Glysennid tablets, 40
Gonorrhea, 20
Grazes. See Wounds
Group psychotherapy, 166

H

Hangover, 60
Head, injury to, 68–69
Head, arm, and trunk rotations, 207
Headache, 60–61

tension, 159
Healthy, staying
  basic needs, 127–34
  caloric value of common foods,
    144–48
  disease prevention, 137–40
  and exercise, 167–74, 205–22
  how things go wrong, 134–37
  and obesity, 140–44, 149–52
  obtaining right balance for, 180–
    81
  and proper nutrition, 152–54
  and regular check-ups, 180
  and smoking, 154–58
  and stress, 158–67
Heart and lung exercises, 213–18
Heart attack/disorders, 137, 139
  care of patient after, 120
Heartburn, 62–64
Hematuria, 99
Hemorrhoids, 20
Herd instinct, 128
Hiccups, 62
High blood pressure, 27
Hoarseness, 62
Hodgkin's disease, 59
Holger-Neilsen method of
  resuscitation, 33–34, 48
Home, nursing care at, 5–6, 107–25
Home physical therapy, 110–11
Hypothermia, 53
Hysteria, 164

I

Ileostomy, care of patient after, 120
Illnesses, causes of, 134–37
Indigestion, 62–64
Infectious hepatitis vaccination, 191
Inflammation, 64–65, 108–10
Inhalants, 10–11, 76
Injuries, treatment of, 65–72
Insect bites, 23–24
Insomnia, 90–91
Instincts, 128–30
Intercourse, pain on, 83
Intermittent claudication, 85
Irritation, 72–73

Itching, 72–73

J

Jaw, fractured, 69
Jogging, 171–74
Joints, pain of, 83–84

K

Kaolin, 9, 10, 45
  poultice, 31
Kaopectate, 9
Kidneys, 99

L

Laryngitis, 62
Laxatives, 11
  use of, 38–40
Leg
  exercises for, 211–12
  fractures of, 72
Legionnaire's disease, 136–37
Leisure activities, and accident
    prevention, 188–89
Leukemia, 59
Librium, 166
Light-headedness. *See* Dizziness
Linaments/balms, 64–65
Lorazepam, 166
Lozenges, 10
Lumps, 73
Lymphadenopathy, 59

M

Malaria vaccination, 191
Medicine chest, contents of, 7–11
Menopause, 73, 74
Menorrhagia, 73
Menstruation, 29
  problems, 73–74, 159
Mental disorders. *See* Emotional
    disorders
Miscarriage, 29
Mobility exercises, 205–7
Monoamine oxidase inhibitor drugs,

166
Mouth
  bleeding in, 27–29
  ulcers of, 96
Mouth-to-mouth resuscitation, 31–
    33, 48
Mumps, 83
Murray, Al, 168
Muscles, pain of, 83–84

N

Nasal speculum, 27
Nausea, 60, 101–2
Neck, pain of, 84
Nervous dyspepsia, 63
Nervousness. *See* Emotional
    disorders
Nocturia, 99
Nose
  bleeding from, 27
  preparations for, 11
  running, 75–76
Nursing care
  for bereaved person, 124–25
  for chronically ill or disabled, 121
  for dying patient, 122–24
  for mentally ill patient, 120–21
  for patient after
      colostomy/ileostomy, 120
  for patient after heart attack, 120
  for patient after
      operation/childbirth, 119–20
  for patient in bed, 112–16
  for patient in cast, 119
  for sick child, 117–18
  general, 107–8, 107–11
  obtaining medical help, 111–12
  physical therapy, 110–11
  taking pulse, 108
  taking termperature, 108
Nutrition, proper, 152–54

O

Obesity, 140, 142–43, 149–52
Obsessional neurosis, 164
Olive oil, 11

Operation, care of patient after, 119–20
Ophthalmologist, 54
Optometrist, 54
Osteoarthrosis, 80
Osteomyelitis, 80
Otitis media, 49
Otoscope, 26, 44
Over-the-counter drugs, 5–6
Overeating, 22
Overweight
  concern over, 142
  and drugs, 151–52
  and exercising, 150–51
  how to lose, 143
  and proper nutrition, 144–48, 149, 152–54
  reasons for, 142–43

P

Pain, 76–78
  abdominal, 79–80
  anal, 20
  of back, 80–81
  in breathing, 34–35
  of chest, 81–83
  of ear, 49
  of eye, 53–56
  of face, 83
  for person who is dying, 123
  generalized, 78–79
  headache, 60–61
  on intercourse, 83
  of joints and muscles, 83–84
  of neck, 84
  of shoulder, 84
  in swallowing, 91–92
  threshold, 76
  tolerance for, 2
  on urination, 99–100
  on walking, 85
Paleness, 85
Palms forward curl, 219
Palpitations, 85–86
Parapectolin, 9
Paratyphoid vaccination, 191

Parkinson's disease, 96
Patient, being good, 202–3
Pedestrians, and accident prevention, 187
Peptic ulcers, 9, 63, 79
Peritonitis, 79
Pharmacist, getting help from, 6
Pharyngitis, 41, 91–92, 93
Phobias, 163–64
Pleurisy, 35
Pneumonia, 41, 137
Poise, importance of, 174–79
Poisoning, 7–8, 86–87
  prevention of, 184–85
Poliomyelitis vaccination, 191
Polymenorrhea, 73
Posture, 174–79
  exercises for, 177–79
  importance of, 174
Presbycusis, 44
Press behind neck, 219
Pressure dressing, 25–26
Preventive medicine, 137–40
Proctitis, 20
Proctoscope, 21, 39, 45
Prognosis, 202
Progressive press-ups, 208–9
Prostrate gland, 99
Pruritus, 20, 72–73
Psychoanalysis, 166
Psychosomatic illness, 159
Pulse, taking of, 108

R

Rabies, 22, 191–92
Rashes, 87–88
Recovery position, 14, 15, 41, 98
Rectal spasm, 20
Rectum, 29
  inflamation of, 20
Relaxation, importance of, 174–79
Resuscitation, 14, 31–34
Rheumatism, 34, 64, 83–84, 84
Rhinorrhea, 75–76
Rowing, 219
Running on the spot, 215

S

Salt
  gargle, 10, 92, 93
  solution for sore eyes, 11
Saunas, 152
Scalds, 36–38
Self-treatment, 5–6
Senekot, 40
Senna, 40
Shingles, 82
Shivering, 94–95, 95–96
Shock, 71, 85, 88–89, 106
  prevention of, 89–90
  treatment of, 14, 25, 29
Shoulder, pain of, 84
Side bends, 206, 220
Sigmoidoscopy, 21
Silvester method of resuscitation, 34,
    48
Sinusitis, 83
Sit-ups, 222
Skin
  disorders, 159
  preparations for, 10
Sleeplessness, 90–91
Smallpox vaccination, 190
Smoking, 154–55
  stopping, 155–58
Snake bite, treatment of, 24–25
Sore throat, 91–92
Sores, 96–97
Spinal arthritis, 80
Spinal injuries, 69–70, 80–81
Splinters, 92–93
Sports, benefits of various, 169–70
Spot reducer, 152
Sprains, 64–65, 66–67
Squats, 220
St. Vitus' dance, 96
Sterilization of instruments, 109
Stings, treatment of, 22–25
Straight arm pullover, 222
Strains, 64–65, 66
Strength exercises, 208–13
Stress, 158–67
Stroke, 139
Suffocation, 31

prevention of, 184
Sunburn, 38, 189, 194
Suppositories, 21, 40
Swallowing, 93
  pain on, 91–92
Sweating, 93–94
Swelling, 94
Swimming, and accident prevention,
    188–89
Symptoms, 1–4
  description of, 199–200
  use of over-the-counter drugs to
    treat, 6
Syncope, 46
Syphilis, 59, 96, 97

T

Temperature, 94–95, 194–95
  and convulsions, 40–41
  taking of, 108
Temporal arteritis, 83
Tetanus vaccination, 191
Throat, sore, 10, 91–92
Thyroid disorders, 22, 96
Tonsillitis, 60, 91–92, 93
Tourniquet, use of, 26
Tracheitis, 41
Train travel, 193
Trembling, 95–96
Trichomonas, 101
Trunk, knee, and hip bends, 206
Tuberculosis, 80
Turkish baths, 152
Twitching, 95–96
Tylenol, 9, 60
Typhoid vaccination, 191

U

Ulcers, 96–97
Unconsciousness, 14, 46, 97–98
Urethra
  bleeding from, 29
  discharge, 98–99
Urinary conditions, 29, 99–100
Urination, pain on, 99–100

Urticaria, 72

V

Vacation
  and health luggage, 192–94
  preventive care for, 189–95
Vaccinations, 189–92
Vagina
  bleeding from, 29
  conditions of, 100–101
  discharge, 159
  and menstrual problems, 73–74
Valium, 166
Varicose veins, 96
Vertigo, 46
Vibrating machine, 152
Vocal cords, irritation of, 62
Vomiting. See Nausea

W

Walking, Pain on, 85
Weakness, 102
Weight
  and appetite, 21–22
  guide for proper in men and
      women, 141
  loss of, 103
Weight training, 217–22
Wheezing, 103
Work, and accident prevention, 187–
    88
Wounds, 104
  bleeding from, 25–26
  covering, 14
  first aid for, 104–6
  nursing care, 108–10
  to the eye, 55

XYZ

X-ray, 26, 63
Yellow fever vaccination, 191
Yellow jaundice vaccination, 191
Zinc oxide cream, 10, 21